Shaping Up

Shaping Up

How to Rid Yourself of Sags and Bulges and Reshape Any Area of Your Body in One Month

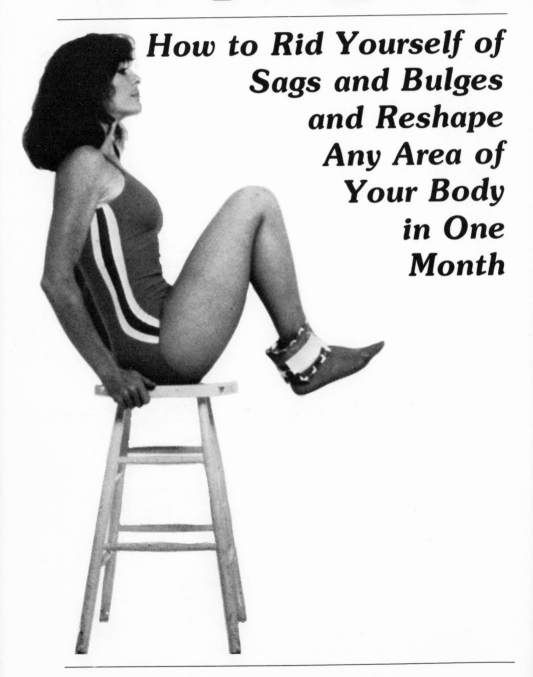

by Sidney Filson

Photographs by Bert Torchia

LITTLE, BROWN AND COMPANY   Boston/Toronto

FIRST EDITION

Recipes appearing on pages 152 to 165 from
Jump Into Shape, © 1978 by Sidney Filson and
Claudia Jessup, reprinted with permission of
Franklin Watts, Inc.

LIBRARY OF CONGRESS CATALOG CARD NO. 80-80704

MV

Designed by Janis Capone

*Published simultaneously in Canada by Little,
Brown & Company (Canada) Limited*

PRINTED IN THE UNITED STATES OF
AMERICA

This book is dedicated to healer
Yolanda Betegh

My thanks and special acknowl-
edgment to William H. Bauther,
M.D. of New York Hospital for
poring over this manuscript to
assure the safety of all my "reshapers."

Ah, Love! could thou and I with Fate conspire
To grasp this sorry Scheme of Things entire,
Would not we shatter it to bits — and then
Remould it nearer to the Heart's Desire!

The Rubáiyát of Omar Khayyám

Contents

Shaping Up

Introduction

Meet Ellen

Ellen Before

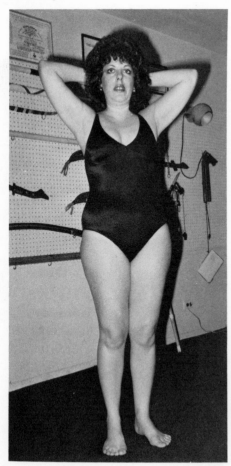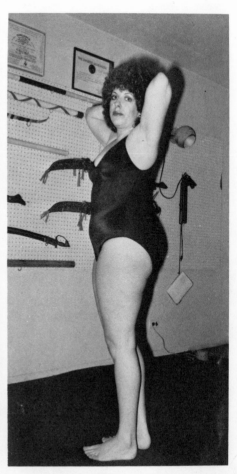

This book is for those who fight the small battle of the bulge, such as the basically fit exerciser who has a pocket or two of fat that won't go away or the dieter who approaches normal weight, but continues to hold areas of fat or flab. It is also for people more than ten pounds overweight who are willing to go on a diet along with this program.

Let's take a look at just one such person . . .

I first saw Ellen standing at the edge of a Y pool. I was swimming in the pool, thinking about writing this book and wishing I had a subject to reshape and photograph. I glanced up and there she was. "Perfect," I thought, "just what I need." She bulged in the places most people do, in the areas that are frustrating because there seems to be no way to remedy them.

I watched her putter about in the pool and when she finished, I followed her into the locker room. I introduced myself as an instructor (I teach jump rope, self-defense, and body-shaping at that Y) and asked, "How would you like to have a beautiful figure in one month?" I held my breath, half expecting her to tell me to mind my own business.

"How? When do I start? What do I have to do?" she asked excitedly.

And with high enthusiasm, Ellen embarked on her reshaping program. She was carrying an extra twenty-three pounds. So in addition to an exercise program, she committed herself to an 80 percent raw-food diet that included lots of sprouts, vegetable juices, and fruit meals.

As with most people who are overweight, Ellen's problem with food was not that she ate too much, but that she consumed all the wrong things. We had one funny food session at my home where I got Ellen to taste all sorts of foods that were new to her. It turned out she liked almost all of them and didn't mind giving up the uglifying foods "because the substitutes are so good."

Then we embarked on the physical program. Ellen was not exactly a jock, but she certainly was game. Teaching her to use weights for body-shaping should have been recorded as a comedy routine. She could hardly heft the small amount of weight, but determinedly wisecracked her way through the first session. She promised to do her daily workout without fail and to increase repetitions — the number of times she did each exercise — steadily.

Ellen chose to reshape three areas of her body: her chin, stomach, and upper thighs. Considering her weight, this meant a lot of reshaping. I explained she'd have to work like crazy and change her entire life-style in order to come in shape by the one-month deadline. She agreed and embarked on my "booster program," as well as diet and weight work.

Ellen became "Miss Game" at the Y and chose racquet ball as her favorite booster. Once a week she attended my women's self-defense class. She improved her swimming capabilities and took to the flutterboard to aid her leg reshaping.

Ellen attracted a lot of attention at the Y. Amazed members watched her speedy transformation. Her body changed and so did her social life.

You will be able both to watch Ellen's progress through this book and see demonstrated some of the exercises that were so successful for her.

Here's Ellen two weeks into her reshaping program

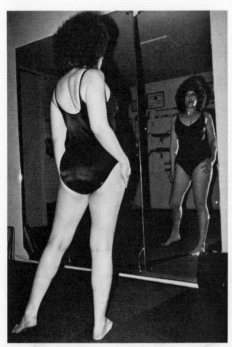
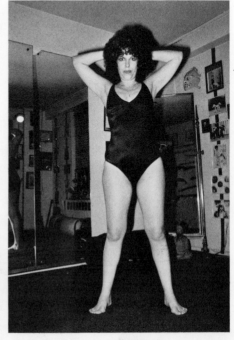

Ellen had some extra advantages that contributed to her reshaping: a terrific sense of humor, an excellent attitude, and an open mind. I never heard a complaint, even though I knew there were times when she ached all over.

So, try to give yourself the same boosts. Laugh whenever possible, don't be afraid to try something new, and stick to your guns. Ellen did it, you can do it too!

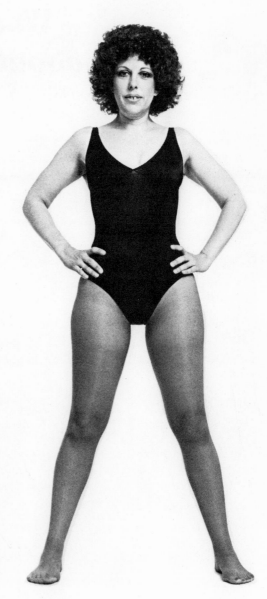

*Here's Ellen almost at the end of her
reshaping program*

Chapter 1

What's Different about Reshaping?

If you've always wanted to have a beautiful body but discarded that goal as impossible, and if your discouragement is due to a figure bulge or slackness that just won't shape up — join the club. Unless you are a rare individual, there's a spot or two on your frame you'd rather be without.

But, don't despair — there *is* a way to dispense with the bane of your existence. It's called spot reshaping and it is the only way to zero in on and repair an offending area.

"But I've tried that and it doesn't work," you may reply if you've been through the fancy health club mill and paid for perfection-promising, beauty-bonus memberships that only made dents in your finances. Or you may have tried the latest miracle diet that took off pounds, but had little or no effect on your particular figure failure. Perhaps you've taken up fitness classes or aerobic exercise — jogging, swimming, or rope skipping — only to discover that while you've been good to your heart and become more fit, the bulge or sag that offends is still unquestionably there.

What I'm talking about is a different kind of *concentrated* spot work. Not a light pass at a problem area, but an all-out war, a fight to the finish with you as victor holding your trophy — a tight, trim figure.

You are capable of smoothing out any bulge or picking up any slack area on your body. You don't have to suffer pain, hardship, starvation, and exhaustion in the process. Neither do you have to spend a lot of money. It is not even necessary to rearrange your schedule to allow for hours of exercise. Ten to fifteen minutes a day is all you'll need to attack your "spot" and accomplish your goal. It's simply a matter of knowing how.

If you will commit yourself totally for one month (two weeks if you can make it through the "torture chamber") and follow this program without deviation, you will solve your problem and learn how to prevent its return. Quickly and surely, you will achieve a youthful, well-toned, symmetrical shape. These methods have proven successful for thousands of people. They will work for you too.

There are plenty of books and methods for allover fitness, but there is not much information on spot reshaping. So, before starting your strategic attack, let's take a logical look at the subject. Here are the most commonly asked questions about spot reshaping and their answers:

What is the difference between overall exercise and spot reshaping?

Overall exercise (also known as aerobic exercise), such as running, jumping rope, and swimming, will condition the heart and build stamina as well as good circulation. Aerobics deal with the intake of oxygen while stimulating heart and lung activity for a time period sufficiently long to produce beneficial changes in the body. Aerobic exercise also improves general health, assists weight loss, and improves muscle tone, but it may not have any effect on small problem areas.

Aren't reshaping and calisthenics the same?

Calisthenics are totally different from reshaping work. Calisthenics are light gymnastic exercises designed to develop flexibility, grace, and coordination. They make for a good warm-up and thereby can aid you in your reshaping. But, done by themselves, calisthenics will have little or no effect on your particular problem spot.

What is the difference between a bulge and a slack area?

A bulge is filled with fat.

A slack area is loose, hanging skin. It can be empty or consist of soft flab.

Why do I have bulges?

Bulges come from bad eating habits and lack of exercise. Everyone has a weak spot, usually where circulation is poorest. Instead of evenly distributing all over the body, fat settles in those debilitated places. It's a rare person who can gain an extra pound or two and not bulge at one point or another on their body.

Why do I have slack areas?

You may have a slack area from nonuse of muscles. A sudden weight loss unaccompanied by muscle toning and skin conditioning is another contributor to hanging flesh. Poor nutrition will also cause loss of elasticity to skin.

I'm over forty. Does that mean it will be harder for me to shape up?

Age has little to do with reshaping. You will be pleasantly surprised, whatever your age, to see how quickly your body responds to intensive spot conditioning.

I'm flabby all over. Can I reshape to firmness?

It will take you too long just with spot work. You'd be better off using swimming or jumping rope as an allover toner and saving spot reshaping exercises for the middle of your body. With that combination, you will quickly solve your problem.

I've been jogging every day and my weight is just right. Why is my stomach protruding?

The midsection is the most difficult spot on the body to reach. Many wonderful aerobic exercises that burn lots of calories and hit other parts of your frame will never touch the stomach. Don't stop your jogging; just add stomach reshaping to your program. The fact that you are running means your circulation is probably very good, and your body will respond and shape up quickly.

Will spot reshaping help me lose weight?

No. Exercise will burn calories, but not as many as we'd like to think. It takes twenty-six minutes of jogging to burn off one ice-cream soda and six minutes of bicycling to atone for one little chocolate chip cookie. An hour of rope skipping only burns three hundred calories. Reshaping does not burn enough calories to make a weight difference. Only aerobic exercise and proper diet will slim you down.

Does it matter how long I've had my bulge?

No. Whether the protrusion is brand new or an old enemy, it will smooth out with concentrated work.

Is reshaping going to get rid of the fat in my bulge?

No. You are going to be concentrating on the muscles underneath the fat. Even when the area looks better and has taken on the shape you desire, the pad of fat will still be there. The only way to get rid of fat is to burn off calories with exercise and by lowering your daily caloric intake.

Will I have to do a lot of different exercises to hit my one problem area?

No. Most often one effective way of moving will solve your problem. Reshaping doesn't have to be complicated. Whenever possible I have given you only one exercise. And that's all you will need to accomplish your goal.

I'm not really out of shape, but my figure is just . . . boring. Can spot reshaping help me?

Yes. To change a boring body to beautiful, one usually has to work the middle. Pulling in the waist can change the look of the whole figure. Or you may be slim but unexcitingly flat. If you need a bit of rounding in the thighs and upper arms, the exercises in this book will help you. If your behind is too flat, the buttocks reshapers will give you a curvier rear.

May I continue to do my exercises during my period?

Yes. Studies based on women competing in the Olympic games revealed that many of them set world records or achieved their own personal best performance during menstruation. Since weight training is a natural tranquilizer, many of these exercises will make you feel better during this sometimes emotional time of the month.

My stomach has been flabby ever since I had my baby. What can I do?

I have worked with many women who were firmly convinced that surgery was the only answer to their hanging stomach flesh. They were delighted to discover how effectively and quickly the methods in chapter seven worked for them. There, you will find a special section for women with stretched skin due to childbirth.

I have a double chin. Isn't that impossible to get rid of?

Of course not. People tend to think that because a bulge is on their head it can't be worked on. Double chins respond to proper exercise very quickly. For living proof, take a look at Ellen's chin as she wends her way through her reshaping program.

Do men and women respond differently to spot reshaping?

Yes, lucky, lucky men. Women naturally hold more fat on their bodies and respond a bit more slowly. Men have fewer places on their bodies that collect deposits of fat. It is rare to see a man with thigh bulge, yet "saddlebags" are the most common problem for women. Most males have one weak area — the stomach. It is the first place to bulge on the male body, but it responds quickly to concentrated work.

Why use weights?

Working with light weights enables you to get speedier results. For instance, you can trim your middle in two weeks spending only ten minutes a day with weights. It would take a half hour a day and a full month to accomplish the same result without body weights.

But won't working with weights give me bulging muscles?

You are going to develop good muscle tone, not bulky lumps that result from "pumping iron." Your aim is to firm and smooth. The amount of weight you will be using would be considered laughably light by any serious weight lifter.

Will reshaping contribute to my health in any way?

Yes, for example, a bulging stomach is more than an eyesore. It means your abdominal muscles are weak and, therefore, your posture is probably poor. As a result, your back is being taxed and will start to complain by means of lower back pain. If your frontal thigh muscles are out of shape, the weight usually supported by them is thrown onto your knees, a sorry syndrome that can end with pain at every step.

All your muscles aid and help sustain other parts of your body. So, when you pull a muscle into shape, you not only beautify that part of your body, but bring it into correct alignment and thus contribute to your health.

Can reshaping change my build?

No. Basic body build is inherited. The length and thickness of muscle fibers are inherited characteristics that remain relatively fixed throughout life.

Somatotyping, developed by Dr. William B. Sheldon of Columbia University, is the procedure for determining what body type you are. According to Dr. Sheldon, there are three major types and each has its own special characteristics:

Endomorph is characterized by a large body, wide abdominal and hip areas accompanied by short arms and legs. Weight is usually concentrated in the center of the body giving a thick or, in the extreme, a "pear-shape" appearance in relation to the upper trunk. There is not much muscle or bone definition and the general appearance is smooth and round. Joints and bones are small in relationship to body size.

Mesomorph is characterized by a solid muscular build. Muscles, joints, and bones are wide and heavy. For men, broad shoulders, massive chest, slim, low waist, and broad hips are characteristic. The upper body has a V shape; the buttocks are heavy and accompanied by large thighs. For women, the muscles are big and firm. The build is generally solid, though not as obviously so as it is for men. The fat tissue (adipose) covering is greater for women than for men in all body types. Good muscle tone is usually apparent in arms, legs, abdomen, and buttocks. The bones and joints are relatively thick and heavy.

Ectomorph. This body type is linear. The bone structure is delicate, even frail. The muscles are slender and stringy. There is little fat. The trunk of the body is short in relation to the limbs. The chest is usually narrow and small.

It is also possible to be a combination of types, though one characteristic type may dominate.

Whatever type you are is with you for life. Just remember that each of these types has its own unique beauty, and reshaping can bring out the best in yours.

My buttocks droop and sag. Is there any way to recapture the terrific curves I once had?

Yes. When you reshape you don't just smooth and firm, you lift. This process is especially noticeable when working on the buttocks. The muscles there are large, and respond very quickly to the right exercise. You can even regain your sexy, youthful indentations.

Can anything be done about small or sagging breasts?

Weight and heredity determine the size of your breasts, which are composed of glandular and fatty tissue. Therefore, exercise will not increase their size. But the chest muscles lying under the breasts will affect the appearance of this area. Strengthening these muscles will tone the chest region, lift, and generally increase the overall chest girth.

What is cellulite and why do I have it?

Since there is a great deal of controversy over whether cellulite exists at all, I'm going to refer to the condition as hard-packed fat. It is not simple fat, but complex lumps comprised of fat, water, and toxins. These ingredients blend together to form a jellylike substance, which lies locked just under the skin's surface. These pockets of "fat gone wrong" act like sponges that absorb large amounts of water, blow up, and bulge out. They result in the ripples and flabbiness you hate. If you squeeze a lump that holds hard-packed fat, the skin will take on the appearance of an orange peel. Plain fat remains smooth in appearance when compressed.

People who hold this type of fat on their bodies are usually large consumers of dairy products, meat, salt, and refined foods. Poor circulation is another major villain. A person who sits for many hours at a time stops the circulation in their buttocks, hips, and thighs and would be a prime candidate to collect hard-packed fat in those areas.

Can I shape up an area that's holding hard-packed fat without dieting?

You can smooth out the lump and cause a marked improvement by means of reshaping work.

Will reshaping get rid of hard-packed fat?

No. Only a special diet combined with reshaping and a unique way of massaging will make any inroads on this problem. For details on diet see chapter twelve. Chapter thirteen will teach you how to massage hard-packed fat areas.

Must I lose weight in order to reshape?

You may be as much as ten pounds overweight and use spot reshaping to obtain an enviable figure. Fifteen extra pounds is stretching your luck, but it's still possible with very hard work. Anything over that calls for weight loss as well as spot reshaping exercises. You would have to go on a program similar to Ellen's, which includes a diet and allover exercise.

Is it possible to make one area on my body larger and another smaller at the same time?

Yes. For instance, you might like to increase your chest measurement, while reducing your thigh measurement. Entirely different muscle groupings are involved, and one area would have nothing to do with the other.

Do the electric spot reducing machines work?

No. Constant use of a vibrating belt will break down skin tissues and leave stretch marks on your skin. The very expensive home machines that attach to your body with electrodes and dispense shocks at intervals are uncomfortable and I have never seen any positive results. Both machines would stimulate a bit of circulation, but you would do that and work your muscles with any sensible movement of the area you want to shape up.

Can I correct my posture by means of reshaping exercises?

Yes. Working the upper body will improve your posture and exercising your midsection will also improve your carriage.

But, after all the work won't my problem just come back?

No, because once you are satisfied with the way an area looks, you are going to learn how to maintain your newfound beauty for life! For specific details on a maintainance program, see chapter fourteen.

Chapter 2

The Magical Month

This chapter will give you hints and tips on how to use the shape-up exercises in this book to your best advantage, so that the next four weeks may indeed be a "magical month" for you!

DO A BODY EVALUATION

The very first step in achieving a beautiful body is to recognize what's wrong so that you can correct the fault. People tend to fool themselves about their shapes. We've all seen friends with a protruding stomach pull in the unsightly bulge for a look in the mirror. There they stand, middle held tight, looking pleased. Then, they turn to the side and pull even tighter on their muscles. They smile lovingly at their lean side view. One friend of mine contracts his muscles like crazy and pounds on his stomach with his fists while gazing into the looking glass: "Pretty good, huh?" He's delighted with his pulled-in image. But, when he's away from his reflection and not concentrating, what a difference! His relaxed midsection leaves a lot to be desired. He's only fooling himself. Don't you do that. Start the right way with a truthful self-evaluation.

Take off all your clothes and stand in front of a full-length mirror. Turn your eyes away from your image and relax. Stand as you usually do. Now, without adjusting your body or contracting your muscles, look at yourself. I know it hurts, but rest assured, four weeks from now you'll be able to do the same self-examination with pleasing results.

Turn around and, using a hand mirror, look at your rear view. Remaining relaxed, bend over, sit, and squat. Take a real look at your body in motion and in various positions. Try to see yourself as others do.

Next, put on a bathing suit. Move and evaluate again. Note

where the edges cut into your flesh. Finally, put on your everyday clothes. Repeat your moving body check.

Now you know the worst. If you have one area on your body that needs work, your program will consist of only ten minutes a day of spot reshaping. If you have two places that need improvement, you'll have to set aside twenty minutes daily.

MAKE A COMMITMENT

Have a heart-to-heart talk with yourself. Promise to follow through for one full month, come hell or high water! Feeling tired or out of sorts is no reason to avoid your spot reshaping work. As a matter of fact, the satisfaction you will experience after completing your task on a day when you're a little down will make you perk up. You'll be proud of yourself and that's good therapy. So, stick to your guns.

Commit yourself to a time. Many people find morning is best. Your energies are highest then, and a bit of exercise will boost your entire day. But, any time, day or night, will do fine. It may be convenient and more fun to pick a time when your favorite TV program is on. I often catch the news and beautify at the same time. Killing two birds with one stone makes this a break in my day I look forward to.

MEASURE YOUR BULGE

If you are going to be reducing a bulge, you might like to measure it so that you can have a before-and-after comparison. Use a standard cloth tape measure and make sure the tape is level around the entire girth area.

Chest — Stand erect and breathe normally. The tape measure should be level around your chest at nipple height.

Waist — Stand erect and be sure to breathe normally. Do not draw in your stomach or protrude it. Men should measure at height of the umbilicus (belly button) and women at the narrowest portion of the waist.

Hips — Stand with your feet together and maintain an erect posture. Measure around the largest portion of your hips.

Thighs — Measure your right thigh. It will probably be the bigger unless you are left-handed. Stand with your feet about eighteen inches apart. Make sure your weight is distributed evenly. Measure the largest part of the thigh.

Calf — Measure your right calf. Use the same position as for thigh measuring, and put the tape measure around the largest part of your calf.

HAVE A MEDICAL CHECKUP

If you have been sedentary for a while, it's best to have your doctor okay your exercise program. The same applies if you have any past history of injuries or illness. The warm-up you will be doing is very light. But, if you are over thirty-five, or have any doubts about the condition of your heart — have a stress test. You can check with your family physician or local medical centers to see who offers stress testing in your area.

Schools and Y's usually offer this service. The test is expensive — prices vary from $100 to $300, but it's worth it in the long run. It is always best to know your exact capabilities.

WEAR COMFORTABLE CLOTHES

Wear clothes that allow total freedom of movement and do not restrict your circulation. Sweat suits are comfortable; leotards, or a T-shirt and shorts, are fine too. Since you'll be doing jumping warm-ups, women should wear a supportive bra or tight-topped leotard and men an athletic supporter.

DON'T EAT JUST BEFORE EXERCISING

Even though your workout routine is not very taxing, it is best not to exercise with a full stomach. Wait at least one full hour after eating. Do not drink a lot of fluid before doing your stint either. You will be more comfortable with an empty stomach, and avoid any chance of nausea.

WORK ON A HARD SURFACE

Many of the reshaping exercises will call for you to stretch out. The floor is best, with a towel, blanket, or a small rug under you to make the surface more comfortable. Don't use a soft support such as a sofa, which will give under you and defeat your purpose. One woman called me long distance: "Not only are your exercises not working (she referred to a magazine article I had written on spot reducing) but my back hurts." Upon further questioning, I found she was doing leg raises on a bed. Of course her back hurt! The soft, giving surface concentrated pressure on her lower back. She stopped working on her bed, and transferred to the floor. That's all it took to stop her back pain and improve the looks of her stomach.

AVOID INJURIES

Always warm up and stretch before you start your exercises.

In the early stages of a new workout program, the chance of injuries to muscles, joints, and ligaments is quite high. I cannot overemphasize how important your warm-up is. Your exercise time will be more pleasant with a properly prepared body. Warming and stretching will also help to avoid any unnecessary muscle soreness.

FOLLOW DIRECTIONS

Place your body in the exact positions pictured and described in the exercise chapters. Follow precisely the prescribed movements, and do not add any you think might be beneficial. The positions are tailored for maximum impact on your specific problem area, so, make sure you do not deviate from them at all.

CONCENTRATE

Put your mind on the spot you are working on. Work slowly. Try to cultivate smooth movement. The *quality* of your reshaping work is important. So, focus on the area you are working and feel the response of the involved muscles. Keen concentration and slow work will bring faster results. It may take as long as two weeks before you actually feel tuned in to the area you're working on. But it will happen, and this new body awareness will help you whiz along toward perfection.

USE WEIGHTS CORRECTLY

Since you are going to rely on muscle development to beautify an area, you should become familiar with the principles that apply to the lifting of weights of any size. You are going to increase the strength of the muscle involved in your shape-up by using weight as a resistance. Even if your particular program does not call for the use of a weight, you will be using your own body weight, so, these principles will still apply.

Never move quickly when using weights. There should be no speed involved in your reshaping program. Quick, jerky movements with weights could harm your joints and will do nothing to improve the quality of the exercise.

Lift steadily. Your muscles must be in control at all times. If a weight is so heavy that you can only move it by "throwing" it up at the start of the lift, you must change to a lighter weight.

Use only the muscles involved. If you find your whole body moving along with the exercise, you are cheating yourself. In order to improve an area you must zero in with everything, including your mind. It's tempting to help a muscle that's crying for relief by bringing other muscle groups to its aid. But that won't accomplish your goal. Be careful about your weight work. Monitor yourself.

Be especially careful of cheating when you are lowering a weight. Gravity comes into play here and makes it the most likely reason to give in. So, don't let gravity do the work, and just let your weight fall. Make sure the lowering of the weight takes just as much time as the raising of it.

Use the entire range of motion called for in the instructions. If an exercise prescribes lifting your leg all the way into a right angle to your body, make sure you do so on each and every repetition. Doing some halfway will give you a halfway shaped area.

INCREASE YOUR REPS RAPIDLY

Repetitions (reps) are the number of times you lift a weight or perform an exercise. Sets are groups of reps. If you do ten reps of an exercise, rest for a moment, and then do ten more, you have done two sets of ten reps each. Increase the number of reps in each set as you become stronger, and thereby decrease the number of rests.

You will find a repetition goal for each exercise in this book. You may divide that goal into as many sets as you wish — but increase the number of reps, and thereby decrease the number of sets and rests, each day. If the goal is one hundred reps, and you are not used to pushing the muscle involved, start out by doing fewer reps in small sets. It's going to be up to you to push ahead as the exercise becomes easier. For instance, on the first day, five reps may be all you can do without stopping to rest. That's okay, it's a start. Do five reps, let your muscles relax for a minute, then do another set of five reps. Keep on repeating these small sets, they'll add up. The next day you must push ahead on each set. If you were doing five per set, pick up the count to six. The day after that, add another rep or two to each set.

You may not be able to achieve your repetition goal at first. But if you make "Increase!" your motto, you should reach it by the end of the first week. The sooner you reach it, the faster your reshaping will be accomplished.

It doesn't really matter into how many sets you divide your repetition goal. The point is to always keep the exercise a little difficult. Once it becomes easy, it's time to increase the number of reps in each set.

PUSH YOURSELF: A SPECIAL NOTE TO WOMEN

Most women are not used to challenging themselves physically and are reluctant to continually push themselves further when working out. The idea threw me for a loop at first, too. I would contemplate giving up; "I'm tired, I can't push anymore." But I did push at that point, even if it was only one more rep. And I soon realized that the next session was easier, or that I needed a bit more weight to provide a challenge.

Quite often women come to me and get instructions for spot shape-ups. I monitor their progress and find great improvement for the first week or two. Then a disappointing period follows.

The mystery is easy to solve. Upon investigation, I find that they have not increased weight or repetitions in that period: "Why haven't you pushed ahead?"

"But it's hard," is the explanation.

Well, it's supposed to be hard. *Every workout should have difficulty about it.* Not to the level of excruciating pain, but you should know you've worked. Your muscles should feel tired.

FIND A BUDDY

Whether you're going to take a leisurely four weeks or a snappy two for your reshaping, it will be more fun with a friend. Weight lifters have long known the pleasure of working in twos. And having a companion to work along with will spur you on to greater efforts. You're less likely to complain about pushing a long unused muscle, and you may even become a bit competitive. I have seen group shape-ups work wonders.

If you have a companion, take turns working out. For instance, if your repetition goal is one hundred, do a set of twenty-five, then give your partner a turn. Count as your partner does twenty-five. This gives you a chance to rest. As soon as your friend finishes, it's your turn to start again. Keep going back and forth until you've both completed your required number of repetitions. The two of you may do entirely different exercises; that will make no difference in your joint workout. The only important thing is for each of you to get your count done.

BREATHE PROPERLY

Never hold your breath while exercising. Breathe naturally as you move. You may find yourself falling into the rhythm of your breathing with your movement. If that happens, it will make your workout more pleasant.

DON'T FROWN

It takes many facial muscles to form a frown. The energy that goes into making a grimace would be better directed at the area you are reshaping. So keep a relaxed face and do not show effort with each movement of your weight.

END EVERY WORKOUT UPSIDE DOWN

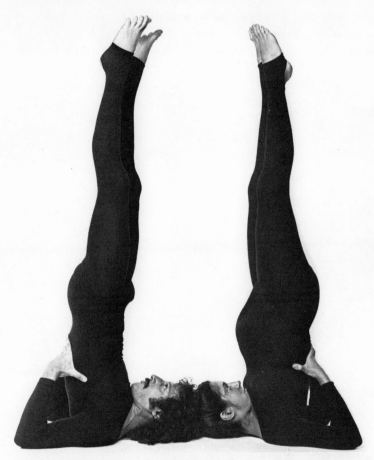

Yogic experts Mark and Yamuna Becker demonstrate a shoulder stand. Yamuna, seven months pregnant, feels women should continue regular exercise throughout pregnancy.

When you're upside down, you send blood to areas that hold fat deposits due to poor circulation. More health benefits — internal organs, such as the kidneys and bladder, take a welcome rest from gravitational pulls. Best of all, inverted postures are nature's little face lift. Just take a look in the mirror after being upside down for a few minutes, you'll happily see the beautifying benefits for yourself.

So, after every workout, reverse yourself for a refreshing finish. If you are familiar with Yogi postures, use the "plow" (also an incredibly powerful tranquilizer), shoulder stand, or a head stand. If you are not trained in Yoga, get instruction before attempting reverse postures so that you do not injure yourself, or lie on the floor and put your feet up above your head on a chair or sofa. The higher your feet are, the more you benefit. A minute or two is adequate.

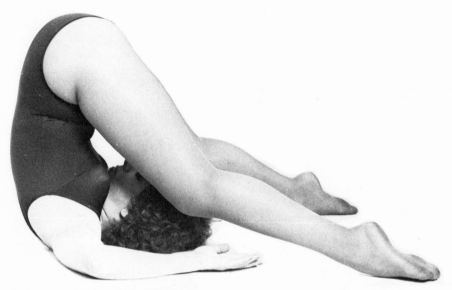

Ellen demonstrates the "plow." This position lets your internal organs rest; you're reversing the gravitational pull.

PLAN TO MASSAGE

Massage contributes to a healthier muscle tone and a better distribution of fat deposits by stimulating and increasing blood circulation in underlying organs and tissues.

If your time is limited, you may just massage the area you are reshaping. But the overall massage is preferable. For complete information, see chapter thirteen.

EXPECT SOME SORENESS

Your muscles should ache during your workouts. If they don't, you had better increase your repetitions or add more weight. This soreness is the first indication that everything is going along as planned. Welcome it. Don't baby yourself at this point! That's why you've got the out-of-shape area. *Now* is the time to push. If you've had your medical checkup, and you have received the go-ahead, do not back off because your muscles feel tired and sore.

That burning feeling is nothing to worry about. As a matter of fact, it's a positive sign. At first, the muscle you are working uses the fuel, muscle glycogen, that is bound into that muscle. But as you continue to work it, the muscle runs out of glycogen and begins to ache. At that point it will start to burn fat.

Dr. William H. Bauther, who specializes in sports medicine, says it's perfectly all right to work through the ache rather than to stop and wait for the pain to die away.

This is the "joyful pain" that professional weight lifters seek. I welcome the feeling when it starts, because I know that it brings me nearer to my goal.

YOU MAY LOOK WORSE FOR A WHILE

There are several areas on your body that will definitely appear more out of shape before they look better. This is to be expected and only means that your muscles are working and changing. In the "Not-To-Worry" sections of some chapters, you will find exact descriptions of how the area will look at its worst. These descriptions are provided so that you do not become discouraged when the spot you are working on suddenly seems to take a turn for the worse. You will have to wait out this period. It usually lasts only two or three days, but, in some cases, it may linger for as long as a week. I have received panic calls from avid spot reducers. "It's getting worse; I'm more out of shape than when I started," they lament. I assure them that's a good sign and try to calm their fears. Sure enough, a few days later, they're back on the phone. "You were right, I look terrific." So, please, don't throw a fit if a bulge seems to be getting bigger or seems to be taking on an even more undesirable shape. It's going to be all right, I promise.

IF YOU HAVE A SETBACK

If an illness or injury prevents you from working out for a while, don't take it too much to heart. Whether your layoff is a week or a month, as soon as you're fit to go back to a reshaping workout, just start with a small number of exercise repetitions again and build back up to your repetition goal. You'll move along rapidly — more quickly than the first time you started.

WAYS TO SPEED UP YOUR RESHAPING

Adopt Boosters

Playtime boosters are sports and leisure time activities that can be used to aid your reshaping. During the "Magical Month" you might as well play in a manner that will compliment your special program. And you might like your new playtime pastime enough to incorporate it into your life-style permanently.

Some of the playtime boosters are quite unusual and may spark your imagination, even if you dislike active pastimes. For further information on common and uncommon playtime boosters, there is a suggested reading list of books in the back of this book. For classes in the Chinese and Japanese martial arts mentioned, consult your Yellow Pages under the name of the specific system.

At-home boosters are sneaky ways to fight the bane of your existence. Sometimes, without exerting any great effort, you can hit the spot you're working on. Making simple changes in a motion you use several times a day can make a great difference in your body shape. You can alter the way you accomplish simple tasks in your everyday routine, and work your weak spot at the same time. For instance, if flabby upper arms are your particular problem, you will be able to work on them every time you scrub clean a sink, wash a window, or polish a car. Just using a circular scrubbing motion, instead of a back and forth one, will speed upper-arm shape-ups.

You will find your particular boosters listed under the area of the body you are reshaping.

The Torture Chamber

The "Torture Chamber" can be found at the end of each area's workout. It is definitely not for everyone. Entering means a super hard-to-do exercise, and you will suffer! "Torture Chamber" movements will tax your endurance and make your muscles scream. So, don't attempt this painful path unless you already consider yourself in the "jock" category, or don't mind being suddenly thrust into it.

Be sure to check with your medical advisor before starting the grueling routine to make sure you're fit enough to undertake it.

Two-Week Half-Time

If you are desperately short of time to whip a neglected area into supershape, "Two-Week Half-Time" is for you. I have had great success with this program when the person involved was being pressured by a job deadline:

Susan was a model. One day she received a call from her agent — she had been selected to do a national TV commercial. The job would mean a lot of money and exposure. Susan should have been ecstatic. But, there was a problem. The job called for her to wear a bathing suit, and she had gained a few pounds on a vacation. The weight had gone to her upper thighs and there it sat. She had been meaning to start an exercise program to combat her new bulges but hadn't gotten around to it yet. Susan called me in a panic, and that's how this two-week concentrated reshaping formula came about.

Susan solved her problem. She followed my instructions to the letter, worked really hard to shape up her thighs, and looked fabulous in the TV commercial.

Since that experience, I have had occasion to work with many people who either didn't have the patience for a month-long program, were gluttons for punishment, or, like Susan, were under the gun to meet a beauty deadline.

Whatever your reasons for participating in this speedy program, make sure you are in the proper physical condition both to work hard and tax your muscles. Check with your doctor.

Here are the rules for "Two-Week Half-Time." If you are overweight, you must go on a diet. You must also:

1. Double up on all exercises, including your warm-up. If the directions call for twenty reps, you must knock out forty.
2. Go into the "Torture Chamber" for every area you are reshaping.
3. Incorporate a playtime booster into your life-style for the next two weeks and work at it. Pick the one that is the most appealing or the most available to you.
4. Work with the required at-home boosters for your problem area.
5. Use the reshaping massage and body oil explained in chapter thirteen.

GET THE RIGHT EQUIPMENT

A minimal amount of equipment is required to use this book, but you should take some care in selecting it.

Shoes

Proper athletic shoes are extremely important. You'll need a good quality running shoe. Look for the one with the *most padding under the ball of the foot.* Since you're going to be up on your toes for your reshaping warm-up, it is necessary that this area of the shoe be well cushioned.

Weights

Read the chapter on the specific area you are reshaping, and see if the exercise calls for the use of body weights. If weights are required, take the time to find the right ones.

Weights come in sets of two. They should fit comfortably on your wrists, ankles, and insteps. You can buy weights in sporting goods and department stores. There are several different types on the market.

One widely sold adjustable weight fits over the foot and laces up like a shoe. It is gold colored, made of heavy canvas, and has pockets on the inside for small metal bars. These bars can be added or subtracted, as you please. Their weight range is from two to ten pounds each. The usefulness of this type of weight is limited since it is only comfortable on the foot and is bulky to travel with. The price ranges from twenty to twenty-five dollars.

Permanently fixed weights are available in two-pound, three-pound, and five-pound sizes. If you are going to purchase weights, I recommend the three-pound size. (That's a total of six pounds for the two weights.) There are two types of permanently fixed weights: one is black plastic and has one-size Velcro closings, which is all right as long as they fit you. They cost from seventeen to twenty-five dollars. The other type is red, white, and blue plastic and has adjustable Velco closings. I like these best because the straps may be shortened or lengthened, so that they can be used in many different ways. They are also the most inexpensive and cost from ten to fifteen dollars.

You can also make your own weights. You'll need six pounds of pennies, or small stones, and a pair of knee-length socks. Divide your fillers into two batches of three pounds each. Your bathroom scale is fine for checking their weight. Make a knot at the heel of a sock. Drop in some weight. Make another knot. Add the same amount of weight. You should be able to make three pockets this way and have enough material left to tie to the remaining toe piece so it will stay around your ankle. Repeat the procedure with the second sock.

These do-it-yourself sock weights won't last too long, but they will give you an idea of what working with weights is like. You might like to try them out before making a purchase.

Jump Ropes

You may want to jump rope as a warm-up. (See next chapter.) If you don't own a jump rope, a clothesline is acceptable. If you wish to purchase one, here's what to look for in ready-made ropes.

Leather ropes cost a bit more, but you'll find them easy to handle and longer lasting than string ropes. Available at sporting and department stores. Price ranges from ten to twelve dollars.

String ropes are fine for jumping. Available at sporting and department stores. Price ranges from six to eight dollars.

Beaded ropes are very heavy and therefore easy to use. They are a price bargain, but be sure to note the construction of the handle. Don't buy a beaded rope with a thin handle. You won't be comfortable holding it for long. Available at department stores, sporting goods stores, and drugstores. Price ranges from three and a half to five dollars.

Warning! Watch out for gimmick ropes on the market. Weighted handles are hard to use. Counter-devices in handles make for an uncomfortable grip and greater expense. Stick with a simple rope and a comfortably thick handle.

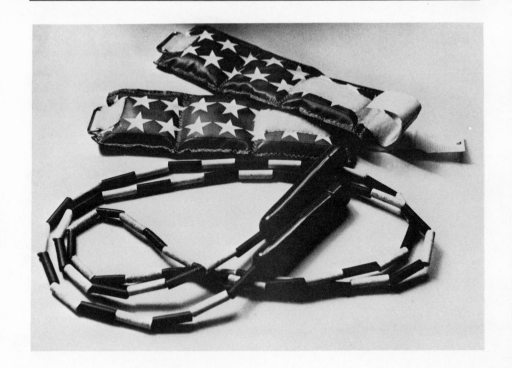

Chapter 3

Warming Up

You must warm up before you undertake any of the exercises in the chapters that follow. The body needs a period of transition to adjust from resting to exercising, and this warm-up process will prevent undue muscle soreness and injuries.

JUMPING

A warm-up must include whole body activity, which raises the muscle and blood temperature enough to produce sweating, but not fatigue. You have your choice of warm-ups. Use one, or alternate between the following two exercises.

Jumping Jacks

One hundred jumping jacks is your goal. You may start with twenty-five, but you should build to your full goal of one hundred by the end of the first week.

1. Jump and open your legs as you clap your hands over your head.
2. Bring your arms down to your sides as you jump and bring your feet together.

Follow these rules:

1. Make sure you stay on your toes all the time you're jumping.
2. Jump lightly. Never pound down. Remember that jumping is taking off, not landing. Think of yourself as feather-light while you do your jumping jacks.
3. Breathe normally! Never hold your breath while exercising. Work at a rhythmic, comfortable tempo.

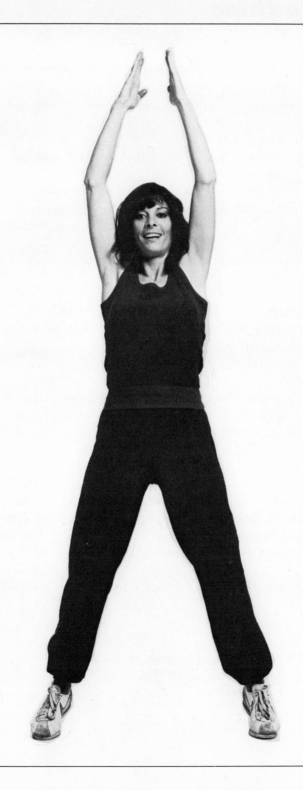

Jumping Rope

One hundred jumps is your goal. As with jumping jacks, you may begin with a count of twenty-five. Just make sure you reach your full goal as soon as possible.

Follow these rules for good form and for the prevention of injuries.

Jump on your toes only.

Wear running shoes and make sure they are well padded under the ball of the foot.

Keep your knees flexed all the time you are jumping.

Breathe through your nose only while jumping rope.

Jump lightly. If you can hear your feet, you're jumping too hard.

Keep your arms still and bent at the elbows. Only your wrists should turn the rope.

The Running Step:

Jump over the rope lightly onto the ball of your right foot. Jump onto the ball of your left foot.

Now right, now left: run in place over the rope, *with no bounce in between.*

You can go slow; you can go fast. Jump lightly onto the ball of one foot, then the other. Keep your knees high, as if you were a prancing pony.

The Doubles Step:

Jump, jump, jump, straight over the rope with *both feet,* landing on the balls of your feet only. Keep your knees bent to absorb any shock. Jump over the rope each time it hits the floor. No bounces between jumps.

These two steps will whiz you through your jump-rope warm-up.*

Expect some soreness in your calves if you haven't jumped rope before.

---

*Sidney Filson and Claudia Jessup, *Jump Into Shape: The Fast, Fun Way to Physical Fitness* (New York: Franklin Watts, 1978) contains more jump-rope steps. See also the suggested reading list.

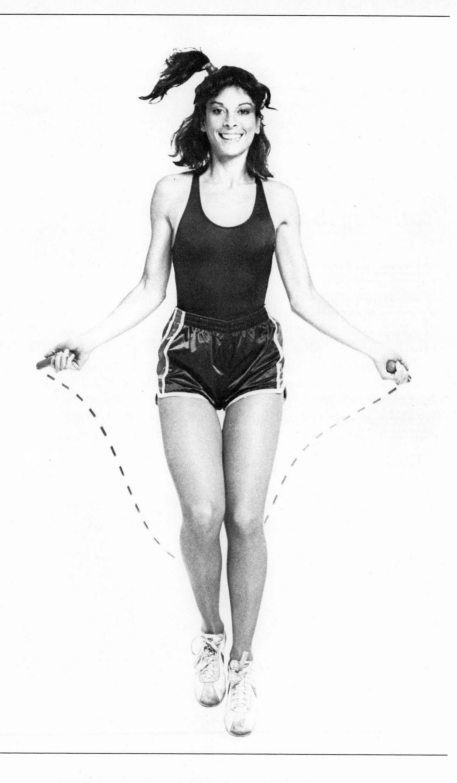

STRETCHING

Now that you've jumped, your muscles are nice and warm. You're going to take full advantage and stretch them. This will help to protect them from injury. Stretching will improve your circulation, posture, and flexibility. The beautiful carriage of the ballet dancer is living proof of the beautifying benefits you can derive from stretching. The lithe movement and peaceful aura of the Yoga practitioner reflect the relaxation and meditative gains of stretching.

Do both of the following stretches as part of every warm-up.

Standing Stretch

With your feet together, legs straight, place your palms on the floor. This should be accomplished with one smooth movement. Be sure to let all the breath out of your lower stomach as you reach for the floor.

If you can't touch the floor at first — no matter. You'll improve each day. Don't push too hard. Let go, and drop as far as you comfortably can. Let your body hang there. Do not bounce! Bouncing is never stretching and will not aid you in increasing your stretch. The weight of your upper body will naturally stretch you. Just relax and let it happen.

Stay in the standing stretch for the count of twenty-five. Come up, take a deep breath, and do one more standing stretch for another count of twenty-five.

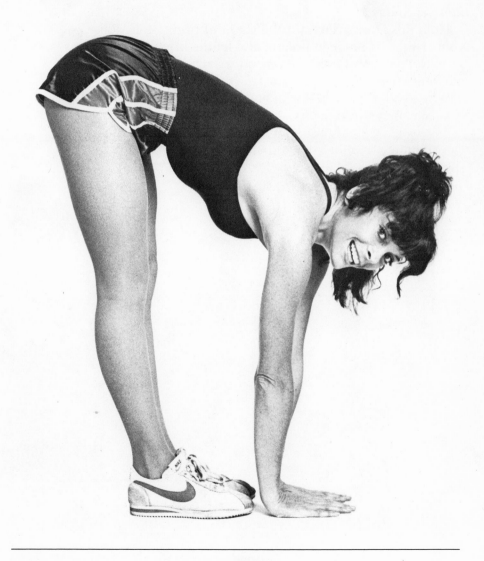

Open Leg Stretch

Next, sit on the floor and open your legs as wide as you can. Let the breath out of your stomach as you bend forward, and try to place your chest on the floor in front of you. Try to grasp your toes with your fingers. The expelling of all air in your stomach is very important to this stretch. You can't bend the body in half if it's filled with air.

In the beginning, go as far as you comfortably can, and just relax. Let the weight of your upper body do its own work. Again, *don't bounce!* Only smooth movement will help you become fully stretched. You will improve more and more each day.

Hold this floor stretch for the count of twenty-five. Raise your trunk, take a deep breath, and let the breath out as you go back down, and hold the second stretch for another count of twenty-five.

When you are finished with your second floor stretch, be sure to close your legs very slowly. Then get up.

Now you are ready for your specific shape-up program. Get right into it while your muscles are warmed and stretched.

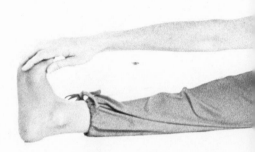

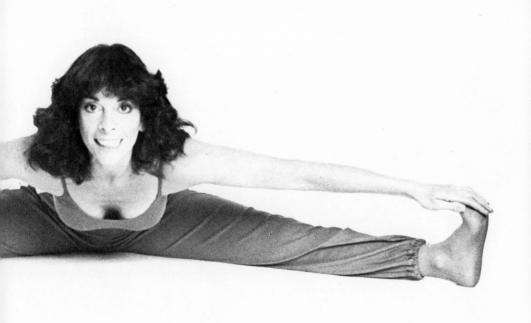

Chapter 4

Double Chin and Neck

DOUBLE CHIN

There's nothing quite as discouraging as being the owner of a double chin: your whole body can be shapely except for that droop twixt jaw and neck. Most possessors of this blight have tried to work it off, but it sits on an area they can't seem to hit with exercise. Well, you *can* reshape this hard-to-hit spot — and without much effort.

I discovered how to beat this particular problem by accident. Responses to a *Family Circle* magazine article I had written on how to flatten stomachs were pouring in. One letter from an appreciative reader caught my attention. "Dear Ms. Filson, thanks for telling me how to shape up my stomach so easily, and another thanks for getting rid of my double chin."

I didn't pay too much attention to her mention of chin reduction until a few other letters arrived saying the same thing. Then, I began zeroing in on double chins and discovered my letter-writing friends were correct.

I had prescribed a raised-head position to keep the spine straight and protect it against injury during the stomach-toning leg raises. That head-held-high posture also caused the hard-to-reach muscles under the chin to work, and thereby beautify the area! So, here's your double chin reshaping exercise, and it's your good luck to get some stomach toning as an extra bonus.

Leg Raises

1. Put a three-pound weight around each ankle.
2. Lie on the floor. Place your hands, palms down, under your buttocks. Make sure you are actually supporting your rear end with the back of your hands. (This is a safety measure for your back.)
3. Lift your head way up. *Your chin should be as close to your chest as you can manage.*
4. Raise and lower your legs without touching the floor. Keep the entire range of the leg raise small. Be sure to keep your chin on your chest. Do not drop your head back to the floor during a set.

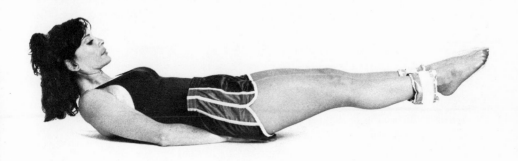

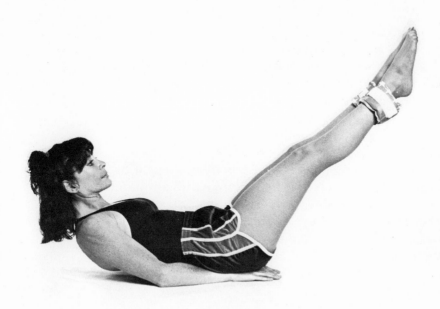

FOR YOUR NECK

Sagging flesh on the neck is a common problem. It starts in the late thirties and gets worse as time goes on. Yet, it is easy to remedy by exercise, although few people aside from weight lifters take the time or trouble to work their neck muscles. Besides making it look better, strengthening your neck is healthy for your upper body. If your neck is weak you are prone to injuries, neck tension, and frequent stiffness. The author of *The Complete Weight Training Book*, Bill Reynolds, credits his strong neck muscles with saving him from a broken neck when he was in a serious motorcycle accident.

To help you firm and expand your neck muscles and take up that extra slack skin, we go to Yoga experts Mark and Yamuna Becker of Serenity Natural Living Center in New York City. Besides contributing to a tighter neck and chin, the exercises that follow will tone the muscles in your face, a special beauty-bonus from an ancient form of body movement and healing.

Do *both* of the following exercises.

Cat Pose

1. Get on all fours.
2. Round your body and drop your head.
3. Inhale deeply into your stomach as you push your chin and buttocks toward the ceiling. You should push hard, creating a deep arch in your back and a strong stretching feeling in your neck. Hold for a slow count of twenty.
4. Relax back into the rounded position and repeat.

Yamuna tells us that this cat pose elongates the body line from the pubic region to the chin. She says it's a wonderful face lift, and that it relieves pressure on and strengthens the lower back. Yamuna, who was seven months pregnant in this picture, also advises pregnant women to do the cat pose for front body tone.

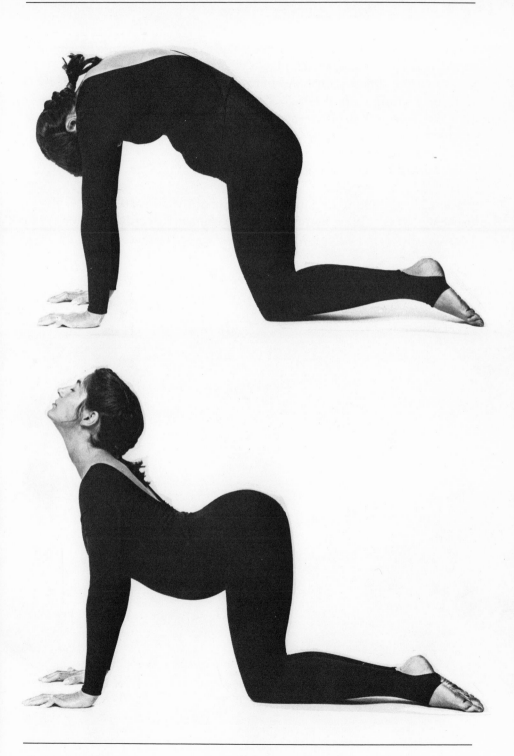

Fish

1. Lie on your back.
2. Come up on your elbows, arching your chest up and dropping your head back.
3. Touch the top of your head to the floor behind, and continue arching your chest.
4. Take deep breaths through your nose, expanding your chest and pulling the air deeply into your stomach. Hold for the count of ten.
5. Repeat, starting from position number 1.

Mark likes the lung expanding benefits of the fish. He advises you to take full advantage and breathe very deeply.

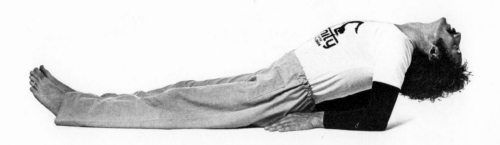

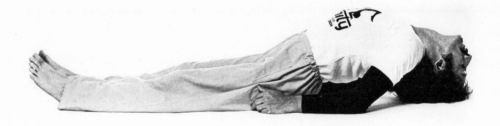

CHIN AND NECK BOOSTERS

Here are some sports and skills you can add to your spare-time program for the next four weeks. Go ahead, have an adventure. Take a "far out" class. Do something you never have imagined yourself participating in. You might as well enjoy yourself as you beautify your chin and neck.

Playtime Boosters

Swimming. The crawl is your stroke. In order to work your chin and neck you do need to use proper water-breathing form. As you turn your head for each timed breath, you exercise the muscles in your neck. To make sure you are using proper synchronization of breathing and stroking in the freestyle (crawl), take a lesson or consult a swim book for instruction.

Hatha Yoga. These breathing exercises and sustained physical postures will teach you how to zero in on all the muscle groupings in your body and how to control them. You will stretch and tighten. I have never seen a Yogi with a loose neck or a double chin. Lots of time spent upside down is also wonderful for your particular reshaping program.

Ballet. This type of dancing will help build a beautiful upper body and a swanlike neck; ballet dancers are not known for sagging flesh. It is a wonderfully controlled body exercise that will leave you relaxed, refreshed, and stretched.

Gymnastics will get the circulation flowing to your uppermost parts. It provides another bonus: the grace and litheness of a cat. Rings, high bar, and parallel bars would be the apparatuses for you, and free exercise the floor work to beautify your chin and neck. The local Y may offer this course. Cosmopolitan areas have private clubs usually run by former Olympic champs.

Hand balancing. This is a two-person hand-to-hand way to shape up your chin and neck. You'll spend a lot of time upside down. This partner pastime will have you indulge in such wonderful techniques as "high front angles." It is a conversation-piece hobby and a supreme workout. Many local Y's have hand-balancing teams and instruction.

Weight training. This is hard work but a solid building exercise for the neck muscles. *Lateral raises* stretch and tone the neck. *Seated presses* are other ways to build your uppermost muscles. In the weight rooms you'll usually find instructors who are willing to work with you. Make sure you are working correctly, and that your body is always at the correct pitch for the area you are concentrating on. Y's have weight rooms and most health clubs have Universal machines which will enable you to "pump iron". More and more women are taking up this form of body training, and they don't have to worry about developing bulging muscles, as nature has provided them with a hormone which discourages bulgy muscles.

At-home Boosters

Isometrics are great to do while watching TV. Here are two that benefit both the chin and the neck:

1. Place both hands against your forehead. Force your head forward against the pressure of your hands. Hold for the count of ten. Repeat at least five times.
2. Place your right hand against the right side of your head and attempt to push your head to the right as your hand pushes back. Repeat with left hand against left side of head. Hold for the count of ten. Repeat on each side at least five times.

Your neck should be singing to you when you've finished. This "at-home" sitting booster only takes a few minutes. To complete the benefits to your chin and neck, go upside down or put your feet higher than your head for a couple of minutes.

FRINGE BENEFITS

The exercises for chin and neck in this chapter will also contribute to the beautification of your shoulders, chest, and back. The leg raises will flatten your stomach as well as contour and firm the front of your thighs. The Yogic fish and cat pose will tone your face.

TORTURE CHAMBER FOR CHIN AND NECK

This neck builder is used by weight lifters to strengthen their necks for hefting large amounts of weight.

Neck Bridges
Repetition goal: twenty neck bridges.

1. Fold a towel to form a pad. Place the pad on the floor and lie on the floor on your back with your head on the pad.
2. Pull your feet up close to your buttocks and arch your body up, digging your head into the pad by tensing your neck muscles. Make sure to arch all the way up so that you are supported by your feet and forehead. Hold for the count of ten.
3. Relax back down to the floor and repeat.

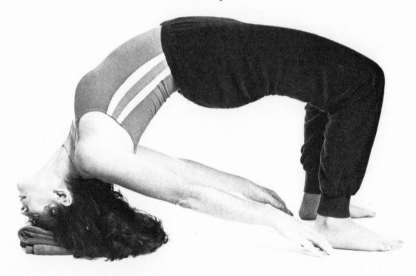

Leg Raises for Chin
Repetition goal: seventy-five a day.

Do your leg raises according to the previous directions given in this chapter, but *move your leg weights from your ankles to your insteps.* This difference will increase the difficulty of the whole exercise. Make certain that your chin is close to your chest and your head is pulled off the floor. You should feel a lot of tension under your chin and in your neck as you do these leg raises.

Do both the neck bridges and the leg raises, then do the upper-arm stretch.

Upper-arm Stretch

Be sure not to skip this last step. You need do only two upper-arm stretches. But if you like the feeling, you may do more.

1. Clasp your hands behind your back, push your shoulders backward, and stretch your clasped hands backward. Hold for the count of twenty-five.
2. Let your arms drop and relax behind you. Repeat.
3. When you have completed two stretches, shake your hands in front of your face as though fanning yourself for a moment. When you have finished, your upper body should feel flushed with strong circulation.

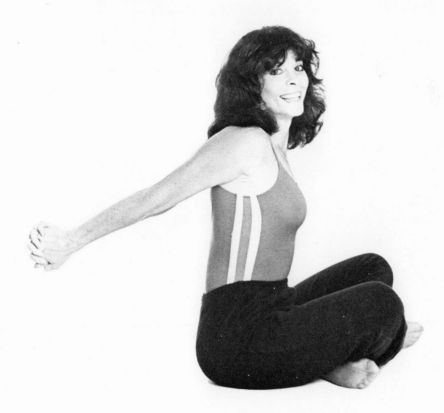

Chapter 5

Upper Arms

My mailbox is always filled with requests for upper-arm toners. "Please help me, the flesh is sagging on my upper arms." "I'm in terrific shape from my waist down, but my arms are flabby." All complaints from *women*. I've never had a male lament an upper-arm problem. Why are women's upper arms out of shape? Because the entire upper body of the majority of women is weak.

In her book, *Getting Strong: A Woman's Guide to Realizing Her Physical Potential,* Kathryn Lance says that in order for the military academy at West Point to admit women cadets, the standards for physical fitness had to be lowered. None of the female applicants could meet the requirements for pull-ups or push-ups. Out of one hundred twenty-seven applicants, only one was strong enough to pass the minimal requirements for men. All the rest displayed an underdevelopment of upper-body strength. Sue Peterson, the women's self-defense instructor at the Point, was amazed because many of this particular group of females were varsity high school athletes. Their schools had considered them physically fit. But, they fell short whenever they had to support their own body weight. When females began to test for fire department and police jobs, the same upper-body weaknesses became apparent.

Are women naturally weaker than men in the upper portion of their bodies? "No," says Dr. Stauffer, director of West Point's "Project Summertime," which carefully monitored the difference between men and women cadets. "There is little limit to a woman's physical potential, but it's just impossible to change the first seventeen years of someone's life in one summer."

Dr. Stauffer refers to the "dainty little flower" image cultural conditioning instills in young girls. It teaches us that it's not necessary for women to be strong. Because of this bias, strength-building exercises for girls are totally excluded by schools in physical education programs. The boys do pull-ups and push-ups, climb ropes, and learn to heft weights. The "ladylike" programs for girls emphasize stretching, posture, and balance. In team activities, the boys are taught to push themselves to the limit, while the girls are allowed to back off when they've had enough. It's still a practice to excuse girls from gym classes when they are having their period, whether they feel ill or not.

The programs at West Point now call for women cadets to be pushed just as hard as the men. And that's what you're going to have to do. Push hard — to beautify your upper arms, *and be healthy.*

You see, hanging flesh on your upper arms is an outward sign of top-body deterioration. This process is not going to stop with some loose skin or a collection of fat. What follows next is a general breaking down of the upper body. Rounded, stooping posture, often called "widow's hump," is a direct result of weakness in top-body muscles. Arthritis in the shoulder joints is another painful reminder that circulation never ranged through that area.

So, as you do your reshaping work, you are going to build upper-body strength. If you find the courage to enter into the upper-body "Torture Chamber," you'll be doing yourself a big favor.

The following exercises will reshape your arms between armpit and elbow. You will need three-pound body weights to work your upper arms. As soon as you finish your warm-up, do all of the following exercises.

Palm Pushes Out

You may start with less. If you can handle only ten on the first day, don't worry, just build steadily — push for twelve on your second day. Try to reach fifty in a week or ten days.

Stand with your feet spread apart at shoulder width for balance. Make sure to keep your knees slightly bent all the time you are working. Breathe normally. Work smoothly. Keep your shoulders back.

1. Put three-pound body weights on your wrists.
2. Hold your hands, palms up, at rib height.
3. Push your right hand forward, heel first, then pull it back into rib-height position as your left hand comes forward.
4. Continue to alternate hands, pushing your right, then your left palm heel forward for a count of fifty (twenty-five for each hand).

This exercise will have both of your arms moving at the same time, one going out as the other comes back.

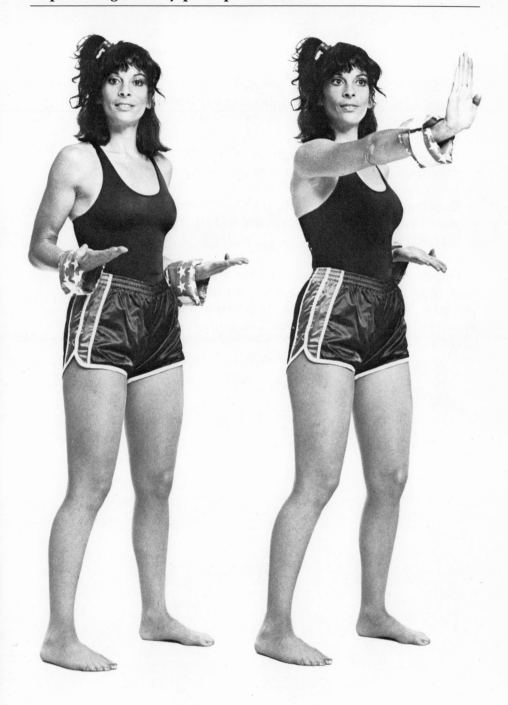

Palm Pushes Up

Stand in the same position as for palm-pushes-out exercise with your feet spread shoulder width and your knees slightly bent.

1. Place three-pound body weights on your hands, as shown in the photograph.
2. Hold your hands, palms up, at your ribs.
3. Push your right hand straight up above your head, heel first, then pull it back into rib-height position as your left hand goes up.
4. Continue to alternate hands, pushing your right, then your left palm heel up for a count of fifty (twenty-five on each hand).

This exercise will have both of your arms moving at the same time. This will tire your arms, but that's exactly what you want. Welcome the feeling. It means you are on your way to shapely upper arms. Now immediately do upper-arm stretches.

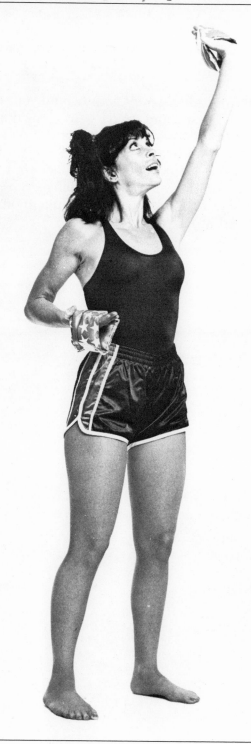

Upper-arm Stretch

Be sure not to skip this last step. You need do only two upper-arm stretches. But if you like the feeling, you may do more.

1. Sit down on the floor, clasp your hands behind your back, push your shoulders back, and stretch your clasped hands backward. Hold for the count of twenty-five.
2. Let your arms drop and relax behind you. Repeat.
3. When you have completed two stretches, shake your hands in front of your face as though fanning yourself for a moment. When you have finished, your upper body should feel flushed with strong circulation.

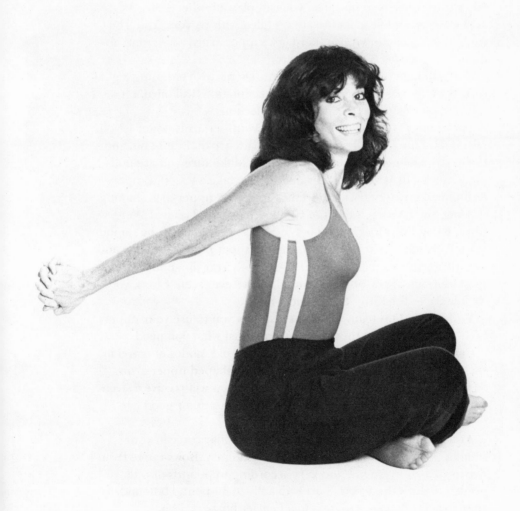

UPPER-ARM BOOSTERS

If you're really serious about the next four weeks of work on your upper arms, you'll change the way you play and accomplish everyday tasks. Here are your best bets.

Playtime Boosters

Frisbee. This is one of the most popular outdoor recreations. Since the frisbee is so portable, you can play anywhere. Streets, parks, yards, and beaches are always filled with players. You'll be using the muscles of your upper back, upper arms, wrists, and abdomen. *Be sure to play with both hands.*

Golf will help tone your upper arms. Do try to avoid using a golf cart. Walking is good for your overall circulation, will burn a few calories, and help make dents in fat collections.

Swimming. When working for shapely upper arms, water is your friend. Use the freestyle (crawl) or the backstroke. Best of all, and the most grueling, is the butterfly stroke. Make sure you are pulling water hard! If your form is not terrific, take a lesson. Proper technique in the water is important for proper upper-arm shaping.

Kung Fu. There is a form of Chinese martial arts called Wing Chun Kung Fu. This particular system was practiced by the famous master, Bruce Lee. It involves using the upper body in strange and beautiful patterns that build mind and body coordination, and the most glorious upper-body definition I have ever seen. Check your Yellow Pages for Kung Fu instruction.

Volleyball. This team endeavor requires you to use your upper body in reaching and throwing patterns. Just what you need.

Canoeing and kayaking. These centuries-old modes of travel in the wilderness will contribute to beautifully shaped upper arms. Along with enjoying the beauties of nature you will receive a strenuous upper-body workout. You must be in a state of good cardiorespiratory fitness for this sport.

Archery. This ancient sport calls for muscular force in your shoulders, upper and lower arms, and abdomen. Bows range from five to six feet in length, and vary according to pounds of pull needed to draw the arrow. Start with a 25- to 30-pound bow and, as your strength builds, progress to a heavier bow.

Martial art weaponry. You can learn to wield a staff a la Robin Hood in Sherwood Forest. *Bo-Jutsu* is the name of this skill, and your upper arms will benefit from the very first day of practice. The Okinawan art of swordsmanship includes learning to use double blades and *sais* (three-pronged swords used two at a time). *Kendo* is the Japanese sportive version of swordsmanship and involves using a mock sword called a *shinai.* This exciting sport calls for constant use of the arms, and chases fat deposits away. All of these skills promote beautiful upper-body definition and are better for you than learning to use one sword, which promotes uneven upper-body development. Look in your Yellow Pages under Karate or Martial Arts for instruction in these unusual boosters.

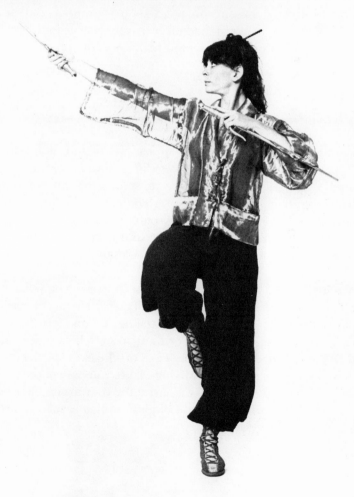

Medicine ball. This grueling little game will require all the strength your arms have. The ball weighs enough to make you exert your catching and throwing muscles. Warning! Improper use of a medicine ball could cause you to pull muscles and ligaments. Get some instruction (in the weight room of your local Y) if you have never indulged before.

Heavy bag workouts. One needn't climb into the boxing ring or enter karate competition to train on a heavy bag. Punching a heavy bag is a wonderful sport for upper arms. If you're female and just starting, you'll find lots of advice from the regulars at the Y. Make sure you tape your hands properly and use gloves.

Weaving. Working at a loom is an artistic hobby that brings relaxation and upper-arm tone. Some Y's sponsor courses, and embroidery shops have materials and offer private instruction.

Speed-bag punching. A great mind-body coordinator and wonderful upper-arm beautifier.

At-home Boosters

Gardening. You can improve the appearance of your home and your upper arms at the same time. Weeding, mowing the lawn, clipping hedges — just what you need for improving arm contours.

Circular scrubbing. I'm sure you wash out a sink during the day or clean a floor. If you've been hiring someone to clean your car, try it yourself. Whenever possible, move your arms in circles. This motion will contribute more to arm shaping than up-and-down motions.

Reach high. *Now* is the time to clean that cupboard you've been meaning to get to for the last six months. The top shelves of every closet await your attention. If you dust ceilings with a mop, do it now. Take advantage of every opportunity to stretch your arms up.

Old-fashioned food preparation. Turn off the electric mixer. Start baked foods from scratch. Mixing makes you use concentrated circular motions that are wonderful for your arms. Alternate right and left hands when mixing. Dough kneading is another arm bonus within food preparation.

NOT TO WORRY

As you are fighting fat off your upper arms, a day will come when the whole area looks worse! You will panic and think you are ruined forever. Don't worry, this period will last from two days to a whole week. It's different for each individual. As the area you are working on goes through changes, it will look bulkier and lumpier just before it looks wonderful. Stick through this period; it forecasts beautiful upper arms.

FRINGE BENEFITS

The exercises for your upper arms will also contribute to the healthy development and shaping of your chest and back. Upper-arm boosters will also aid your entire body.

TORTURE CHAMBER FOR UPPER ARMS

Welcome, brave soul. Prepare to work. Remember, *add* this grueling upper-arm exercise to your palm-heel pushes.

Pull-ups
Repetition goal: thirty pull-ups per day.

Use two grips. Do fifteen pull-ups with fingers facing you and fifteen pull-ups with fingers facing away from you.

Chinning bars are best for doing pull-ups in the house. I've found that the best place to put one is in the doorway to the kitchen. Then you can make a rule — so many pull-ups to enter the kitchen and so many to get back out.

This is an extremely difficult exercise, and it may take you quite a while to even accomplish one pull-up.

Place the chinning bar so that your hands can reach it without your having to jump up. Stand directly under the bar, grip it firmly, and pull. The object is to get your chin above the bar. Don't jump up to it. That won't accomplish your goal. Use rather a steady pulling motion on your way up and a slow lowering one on your way back down. Don't touch the floor between pull-ups (once you can do more than one). You can bend your legs at the knees and keep them up behind you so they don't touch.

Chinning bars may be purchased at sporting goods and department stores. You may also use any overhead device that you can pull yourself up on. I have a friend who uses her children's swing bars for pull-ups.

Don't be discouraged if you cannot do a pull-up. Most women can't. But, don't give up either. Only by trying harder and harder will you ever be able to do it. At first you may only be able to lift your entire body up an inch. But if you continue to try, that inch will become a foot and your chin will be above that bar.

Most men can do pull-ups. Ask a male friend to demonstrate. The ease with which he pulls himself up will spur you on and be a good image for you to think about as you struggle by yourself.

I tell my students to think about pull-ups in this way: you're only holding your own body weight. *You have to be able to hold your own weight.* What if you fell out a window and had to pull yourself back to safety?

I have had students call me on the phone to announce they've finally accomplished their first pull-up. It took Ellen about two weeks of trying to do one. You will be so proud of yourself when you can do pull-ups. It will make all the suffering worthwhile. And there is no better arm beautifier.

Warning! Chinning bars come with brackets to secure them to door frames. Make sure you use them. Without these brackets the bar could come down while you are using it. So be sure to avoid any injury, and secure your chinning bar according to package directions.

If you have no place to do pull-ups, you may substitute full push-ups as described on page 85. Your repetition goal would still be thirty a day.

If you have access to a full-size swimming pool, you may substitute the following exercise for pull-ups.

Water Torture for Upper Arms
Repetition goal: ten laps.

Butterfly is the name of your torturous stroke. You may start with a lap at a time and build to your goal.

Chapter 6

Chest and Back

Chest and back problems travel hand in hand. If your front is out of shape, it's a good bet the back of you needs help too. The letters I get asking for advice speak of "bra bulge," drooping breasts, hanging fat on backs, caved-in chests, skinny, out-of-proportion upper bodies — all manifestations of the same top body weaknesses. If you have no muscle tone, of course, your weak back and chest will allow deposits of fat to settle and slack areas to form. It also stands to reason that underdeveloped muscle structure will result in more than cosmetic problems. When your back looks out of shape, you probably have some lower back pain and frequent backaches. More than any other place on the body, the back is highly susceptible to tension pains. There's no way around the issue: to have a healthy, beautiful back, you must work your muscles.

The properly developed human back is beautiful. The female back is finely sculptured by nature. Toned-up muscles will flank the spine on both sides to form an exquisite "hollow." Smoothly contoured, a woman's well-toned back adds much to her grace and beauty. A conditioned male back has long been the sculptor's delight. Large and strong back muscles take on keen definition and ripple with every movement.

The front of your upper body needs strength to be attractive. Women with drooping breasts can radically improve the looks of their chest by building the underlying muscles. Nothing can affect the breast itself, which is composed of glandular and fatty tissue, but still the whole area can be firm and well-shaped. As muscles respond to the proper exercise, the area just above the breasts takes on a desirable, rounded look and the breast itself is lifted. The shoulders straighten and take on appealing contours as part of the reward for the determined upper-body exerciser.

When males have weak upper bodies, their shoulders and chests seem to fold inward in a defensive posture. But their upper-body exercise is quickly rewarded by a well-rounded chest and firm, well-outlined muscles.

Since good carriage makes your upper body look better, I'd like you to become more aware of how you hold your body while you are improving your muscles. Here are some tips to help establish proper posture habits. Keep reminding yourself of them as you work on your chest and back during the "magical month," and they will become automatic.

In a standing position, carry your body stretched upward as much as possible without strain. Try to feel your head and neck centered between your shoulders. Your chest is always the farthest point forward and should be moderately elevated with no strain. Your shoulders should be held back and down, but never tensed. Your buttocks should be slightly contracted, pulled down and under, which will result in the pelvis tilting slightly upward in front. Your stomach should be flat, but not pulled in to the extent of restricting your breathing. Your knees should be relaxed, never stiff. Make sure to always distribute your weight evenly. Your center of gravity is the middle of your pelvic area. If you were to take a side-view picture of perfect, standing human posture, the ear lobe, the tip of the shoulder, the middle of the hips, the back of the knee caps, and the front of the ankle bone all would be in a vertical line.

In a sitting position, correct posture involves basically the same rules for alignment and balance from the head to the hips as the standing position. It is important that there be no space between the back of the hips and the back of your seat. Don't fall into the usual pattern of allowing your hips to slide forward. This common habit creates an excess curvature of the lower spine, and places terrific amounts of strain there. Another rule to remember when sitting, is always to have your knees higher than your hips. When your knees are lower than your hips your poor back has to overarch and strain. This is a good tip for people who spend hours driving or sitting at a desk. I always put a book under my feet while I'm typing.

So, elongate and think tall as you develop your upper body, and get rid of your problem area.

You will need three-pound body weights to do your chest and back exercises. As soon as your warm-up is finished, do *all* the exercises here.

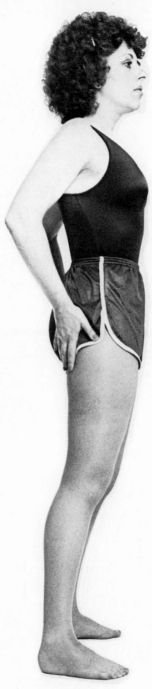

Ellen demonstrates good posture

Half Push-ups

You may start with less, but I want you to build as quickly as possible to the full count.

1. Kneel and place your palms on the floor a little farther apart than your own chest width.
2. Drop your body to one inch from the floor. Make sure your hands remain at chest level, and push back up.

Be sure to breathe normally while doing half push-ups, and keep your back straight! No caving in is allowed.

If you are not used to pushing your weight around, this exercise may seem difficult. It is sure you're going to feel some muscle ache. That's good! Only with such resistance as this half push-up can you help your weak chest. You're going to have to discipline yourself a little. When you feel tired, give it one more try. Push! You can do it!

Repetition goal: fifty half push-ups.

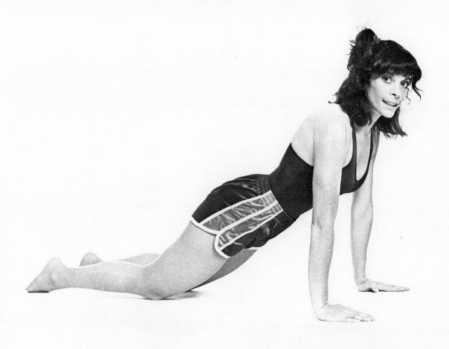

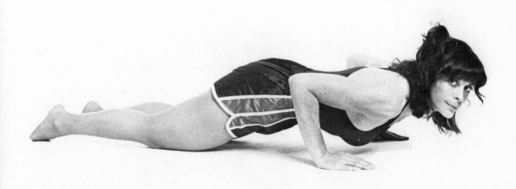

Arm Lift

1. Gripping a three-pound body weight in each hand, stand with your legs straight and your feet comfortably apart.
2. Bend down, keep your arms straight, and very slowly bring your body weights up behind your back and hold for the count of five.
3. Bring your arms down, and repeat. Do not straighten up until you have finished your set.

   Don't arch your back, just keep it straight throughout this exercise.
   These arm lifts have a quick effect on "bra bulge," those pads of fat that women bemoan on their backs. Now immediately do upper-arm stretches.

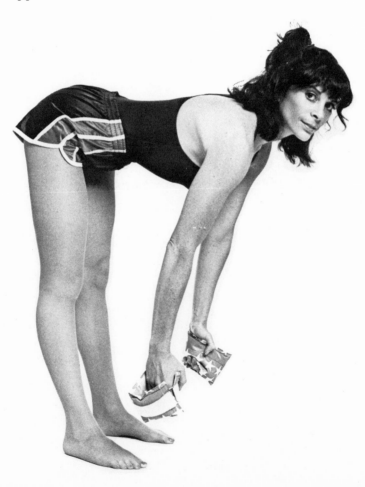

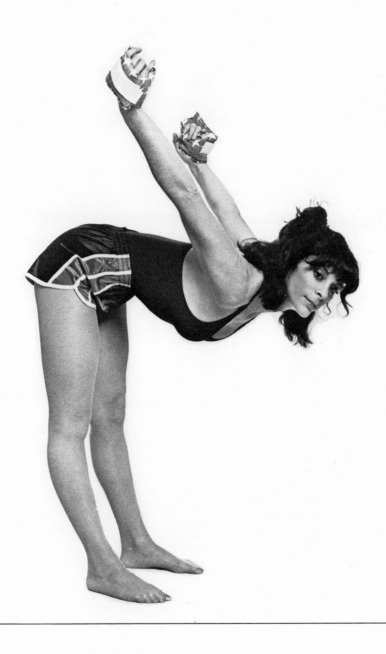

Upper-arm Stretch

Be sure not to skip this last step. You need do only two upper-arm stretches. But if you like the feeling, you may do more.

1. Sit down on the floor and clasp your hands behind your back, push your shoulders back, and stretch your clasped hands backward. Hold for the count of twenty-five.
2. Let your arms drop and relax behind you. Repeat.
3. When you have completed two stretches, shake your hands in front of your face as though fanning yourself for a moment.

When you have finished, your upper body should feel flushed with strong circulation.

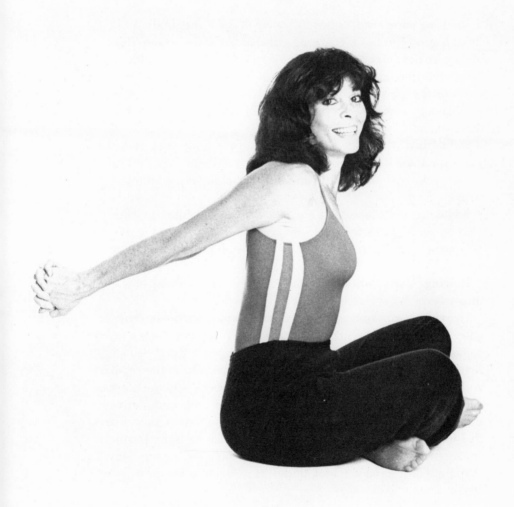

CHEST AND BACK BOOSTERS

Remember, your commitment to the "magical month" included changing some of your recreational habits. Here are your choices. If you make one or more of these fun-filled ways of accomplishing your upper-body shape-up part of your life, you will speed along toward your goal.

Playtime Boosters

Jumping rope involves beneficial use of the upper body. Even though good form calls for quiet arms, don't be fooled into thinking you're not working the entire upper body. Arms, shoulders, back, and chest will shape up.

Throwing games. Volleyball, basketball, medicine ball, frisbee, or just playing catch for a half hour at a time will help tone your upper body.

Swimming. A quick way to tone your upper body. Stay in the water for at least a half hour of nonstop movement. Use the crawl or the backstroke. Best of all, and most grueling, is the butterfly stroke.

Kayaking and canoeing. Enjoy the wilderness while you give your upper body a strenuous workout paddling and portaging. You must be in a state of good cardiorespiratory fitness for these sports.

Rowing. This on-the-water sport requires vigorous use of the upper body.

Heavy bag workouts. One needn't climb into the boxing ring or enter karate competition to train on a heavy bag. Punching a heavy bag is a wonderful exercise for the entire upper body. If you're female and just starting, you'll find lots of advice from the regulars at the Y. Make sure you tape your hands properly and use gloves.

Ballet and karate will both work your upper body and improve posture. Wing Chun Kung Fu is the Chinese system of martial arts that most works the upper body. USA GoJu karate is the Japanese system practiced in America that will give you a terrific top-body shaping. For instruction, look under Kung Fu and Karate in your Yellow Pages.

Martial art weaponry. You can learn to wield a staff a la Robin Hood in Sherwood Forest. *Bo-Jutsu* is the name of the skill and your upper body will benefit from the very first day of practice. The Okinawan art of swordsmanship includes learning to use double blades and *sais* (three-pronged swords used two at a time). *Kendo* is the Japanese sportive version of swordsmanship and involves using a mock sword called a *shinai*. This exciting sport calls for constant use of the upper body and builds beautiful outlines. All of these skills promote terrific upper-body definition and are better for you than learning to use one sword (or one tennis racquet), which promotes uneven upper-body development. Look in your Yellow Pages under Karate or Martial Arts for instruction in these unusual boosters.

At-home Boosters

If you have stairs, you can do **the crawl.** This chest and back booster is one of Bonnie Prudden's favorites from her book *How to Keep Your Family Fit and Healthy.*

Lie flat on the floor at the top of the stairs and simply walk down on all fours, without letting your feet get too close to your hands. Be careful. If your staircase is a long one, start four or five steps from the bottom.

Lawn mowing (with a hand mower), **gardening,** and **hedge clipping** are all valuable home work for your chest and back.

Installing a **chinning bar** is doing your chest and back a favor. Please heed package warnings and use the protective brackets that make the bar secure.

Handstands are marvelous for chest and back development. Simply put your hands on the floor close to a wall, then kick your feet up to that wall. Stay there a while, then come gently back to the floor with your feet. After a while you should be able to do handstands without the wall for support. You may also have another person catch your feet in the beginning.

TORTURE CHAMBER FOR CHEST AND BACK

You asked for it, you got it!

Full Push-ups
Repetition goal: fifty full push-ups.

This exercise will require all the willpower you can muster. If you are female, chances are you can't do even one push-up. Never mind. Get onto your hands and push as much as you can. Even if you only make it one inch off the ground at first, keep at it.

Many women who have trouble doing push-ups ask this question: "Isn't there something else I can do to increase my strength so I'll be able to do push-ups?"

"No" is always my answer. You learn push-ups by doing them. It's like learning to drive a car—you wouldn't practice bicycling to prepare yourself. Your own weight is the perfect learning aid when it comes to doing full push-ups.

Push-ups strengthen the mind as well as the body. In karate this process is called building the "iron will." Armed forces have always

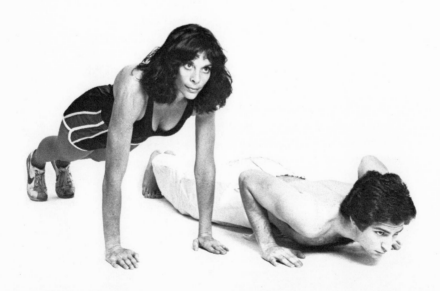

recognized this premise, and push-ups are an important part of all basic training. I want you to build your "iron will," and here's my personal motto to help. Use it when you feel you can't possibly do another push-up. Instead, don't give up, and pump one more for me: "Let's go! Keep going! There *is* nothing else!"

Be sure to breathe normally while pumping push-ups and don't let your back cave in:

1. Support your entire body with your hands and toes only. Your hands should be a little wider apart than your chest width.
2. Keeping your body straight, drop to one inch from the floor, and push back up.

Expect lots of arm ache, but don't let that stop your progress. The discomfort will cease as soon as your muscles get used to working this way.

If you have access to a full-size pool, you may substitute the following for full push-ups:

Swimming
Repetition goal: twenty laps.

Your water torture is the butterfly stroke. Your chest and back couldn't have a better shaping exercise. You may start slowly, one lap at a time, but try to increase steadily and add a lap each time you work out. Work for a straight twenty laps of nonstop butterfly. You'll be the hit of the pool, and your upper body will respond very quickly to this taxing water workout.

If this is going to be your only "torture chamber" workout, do your butterfly exercise at least four times a week. If you are adding butterfly strokes to your push-ups as a booster, three times a week is plenty.

Chapter 7

Stomach, Waist, and Front Thighs

What is the quickest and easiest way to determine if a person is in tip-top physical condition? One glance at the waistline tells the entire story. If the stomach is not flat and hard, its owner is out of shape. If you have a strong abdomen with well-defined muscle outlines, your whole body will appear symmetrical. A tight middle will make even an unshapely top and bottom look better.

In this age of physical fitness, when books on athletics reach the best-seller lists, one would think that loose middles were passé, especially among athletic types. Not so. Unsightly midsections are the most common figure problem for both men and women, including joggers and tennis players. I constantly receive letters complaining about stomachs and waists: "I can't understand it, I jog a mile a day, I do sit-ups, and still I have this spare tire around my waist" or "What can I do to rid myself of 'lovehandles'?" Another typical communique reads, "I'm not overweight, but my stomach sags."

The most discouraged pen pals I have are women who have given birth. They are convinced nothing but plastic surgery will help them, and that last avenue is either too expensive or too scary to be considered.

Well, put a smile on your face. You're going to tighten your middle in no time. I'm going to teach you a winning exercise that hasn't failed yet. When I divulged this sure way to trim middles in *Family Circle* magazine, I received thousands of thank-you letters from men and women who successfully reshaped their stomachs and waists.

But first, I want you to know *why* your stomach and waist are out of shape and why you have an obligation to yourself to have a perfect middle for other than cosmetic reasons.

Your bulging middle is a direct result of the food you eat. Even if your weak midsection showed up after childbirth, it's still a nutritionally based problem. If your skin had been properly supported with vitamins and enzymes and complete proteins, it would have had the elasticity to bounce back to perfection.

You are what you eat. *Meat is heavy.* It will make you the same way. *Bread is soft and pasty.* It will make you the same way. *Dairy products were made for cows,* not humans. Show me a heavy milk, cheese, and butter consumer and I'll show you an out-of-shape waist and stomach. Empty calories consumed in the form of white sugar, white bread, white rice, and pasta, will lie in a band around your waist.

A large stomach is often referred to as a "beer belly," with good reason. "Businessman's paunch" can grow from double martinis at lunch. Wine and liquor not only contain a lot of calories, but those calories have no value to you. Alcohol makes for bloat, not beauty!

I can teach you how to flatten your stomach and have a wasplike waist very quickly. But if you continue the unhealthy eating habits that created your problem in the first place, you will always have to fight this particular problem. The "Magical Month" is a good time to begin making a permanent change in your eating habits. Cut down on animal fats, meat, and dairy products. Eliminate "empty calories" from your diet — alcohol, candy, and foods made from refined white flour. Eat foods made with whole, sprouted grains instead. Increase the amount of raw fruits and vegetables in your daily diet. Some delicious recipes using raw vegetables and fruit will be found in chapter twelve. And while you are reshaping during this "Magical Month," take at least one body-flusher a day. More information about this will also be found in chapter twelve.

The reshaping exercise for your stomach, waist, and front thighs will coordinate your body and breath control — also primary factors in the development of intrinsic energy. The front of your thighs will round to a firm contour as your waist pulls in and your stomach flattens, all as a result of the following exercise.

I first learned this "miracle" reshaping exercise while working my way up to a Black Belt in karate. My instructor was a former marine, and he had a special spot in his heart for "leadbellies." If he spotted a bulging middle on a new student, this therapy was applied.

If your problem is a result of childbearing, *add* the "childbirth-special" exercises to the leg raises and make sure not to skip any of the steps prescribed.

As soon as you complete your warm-up do the following exercises.

Leg Raises

You may start with a lower number of reps per day, but please build quickly to your total goal. This will be a difficult exercise until you get used to using your slack abdominal muscles. You may only be able to do one or two at a time. Don't get discouraged, just do one or two, several times a day. You'll be surprised at how many leg raises you will pile up this way. And since the response to this exercise is so quick, you will soon have plenty of encouragement.

Breathe normally while doing leg raises. How you breathe as you execute this exercise has a lot to do with the result you'll get. If you hold your breath, your muscle won't work properly. Instead, work for easy breathing, and put your mind on your stomach (your waist is going to follow along). Feel the muscle response. Be sure to keep your face relaxed, and don't frown!

1. Put three-pound body weights on your ankles.
2. Lie on your back. Place your hands, palms down, under your buttocks.

   Your hands should be supporting the full weight of your rear.

   Lift your head as far from the floor as possible. Try to touch your chin to your chest.
3. Raise and lower both legs at the same time. Move only your legs, and try not to let your whole frame move.
   You must hold your body in the exact position I describe and demonstrate for two reasons. First is the safety of your back. You don't want any pressure on your lower spine. This position will prevent that. Second you need strong concentration on your abdominal area. Only by keeping your body in this exact position will this reshaping exercise work for you. So be sure not to relax and drop your head back at any time during your leg raises.
   Do not touch the floor with your feet between leg raises. Nor should you raise your legs too high. (A ninety-degree angle would be too much.) Either of these moves would relieve tension on your middle. The whole idea is to keep lots of tension there as you work.

Repetition goal: one hundred leg raises.

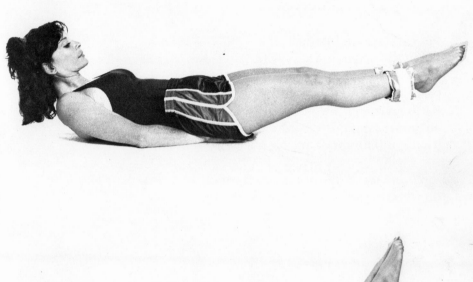

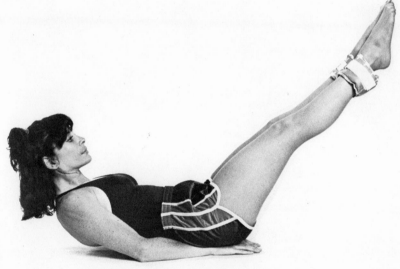

Alternating Leg Flutters

Flutters are interchangeable with leg raises. They relieve boredom and are equally as effective as double leg raises. I usually split my workout into half leg raises and half flutters when I work my midsection. Work sets, they'll fly by.

1. Put three-pound body weights on your ankles.
2. Lie in the same position as for leg raises, hands under buttocks, chin toward chest, head high. Maintain this body position throughout the flutter exercise.
3. Keep your legs low and *slowly* raise one, then the other, in an alternating flutter, for a total count of two hundred (that's one hundred for each leg).

Don't touch the floor between flutters, and keep your legs at the same height as mine are in the illustration.

Repetition goal: two hundred flutters.

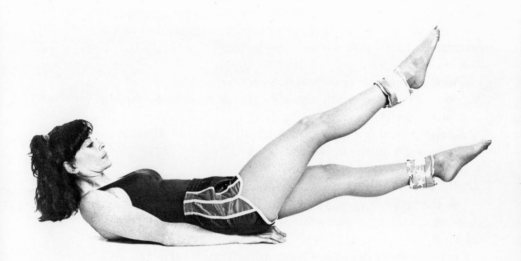

Childbirth Special

These exercises are to be done *after,* not during, pregnancy. If you have given birth recently, be sure to consult your obstetrician to see if it's time for you to start an exercise program.

1. Put three-pound body weights on your ankles.
2. Sit on a stool or bench, or sideways, on a chair. Grasp the seat for support.
3. Keeping your legs together, toes up, and heels toward the floor, pull your knees to your chest.
4. Lower and extend both legs.
5. Pull your legs back to your chest. Repeat.

Use the reshaping massage and body lotion described in chapter thirteen on your stomach *every day* during the "Magical Month."

Add one nutritional skin toner to your diet each day. According to Dr. N. W. Walker, author of *Raw Vegetable Juices,* either of these silicon-rich drinks from nature will make a marked improvement in your skin tone: four ounces of carrot juice and four ounces of green pepper juice or four ounces of carrot juice and four ounces of cucumber juice. These eight-ounce glasses of juice must be made fresh and taken immediately. They cannot be stored, canned, or bottled and hold the vitamins and minerals you need. If you don't have your own vegetable juicer, try your local natural food store; most have juice bars and make to order. A high potency B-complex vitamin supplement, taken twice daily, will also aid in returning elasticity to stretched skin. Remember, your problem has two causes, lack of proper exercise and lack of nutrition. During this "magical month," I want you to work your stomach from every angle.

The sitting pull exercise, combined with lying leg raises, will hit the low part of your abdomen — the hardest area to firm otherwise. This spot responds only to very forceful exercise. But, it will respond; just prepare to work hard. A light pass at your problem will accomplish nothing. As your middle muscles respond, high and low, much of your slack skin will be picked up. The exercise, combined with massage, oils, and nutritional toners for your skin, will rejuvenate this area of your body. It's worked for other women, and it will work for you too.

Repetition goal: fifty sitting pulls added to your leg raises.

All of the reshaping exercises for waist, stomach, and front thighs will cause aching muscles. That's good. Remember you haven't taxed these particular muscles for a long time. Don't use sore muscles as an excuse to not exercise.

After your exercises are done, remember to relax upside down for a few minutes (see p. 25).

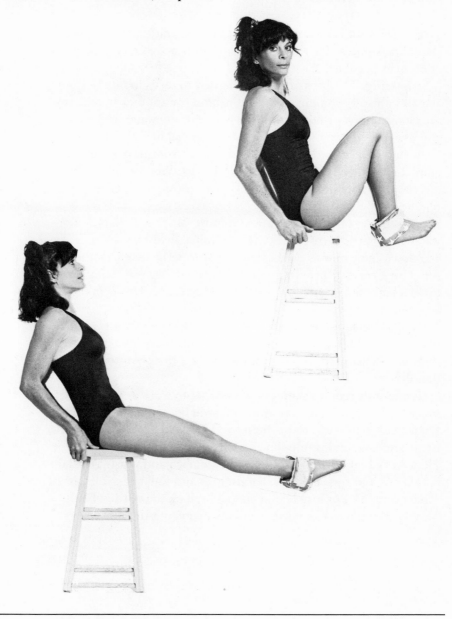

STOMACH AND WAIST BOOSTERS

Playtime Boosters

In order to fully commit yourself to the "magical month," you should pick one of the following leisure-time activities and play at it as often as possible.

Swimming. The backstroke can be used to focus in on the stomach and waist. Each time you reach behind for another stroke, you are elongating your midsection. As you grab the water and pull, you use your abdominal muscles in a beneficial manner. Try to keep your head raised when doing the backstroke to place more emphasis on the abdominal and thigh fronts. You should be able to see your pelvic region as you stroke. Concentrate on feeling your middle as you pull water. The crawl or freestyle can also be used to zero in on your stomach and waist. Make sure to pull the water very hard. That's when the abdominals assist your stroke. If you don't know how to do these strokes properly, take a swim lesson. Using correct form is important in reshaping your body. Work up to a half hour of nonstop swimming each time. Less is inconsequential.

Ballet. Elongation exercises will require the use of your middle muscles. Total body control is called for, and every area of the body is well affected. (Have you ever seen a thick-waisted ballet dancer?)

Gymnastics require center body muscles to work as you cultivate grace and agility. Using any apparatus will boost your middle and front thigh shape-up; rings, high bar, parallel bars, balance beam, horse and box, and trampoline are all exciting ways to reshape. Floor work is also wonderful for your stomach and waist. You'll do backbends and forward rolls, handstands and walkovers, all part of "free exercise." For instruction and clubs, look to your local Y. Most cosmopolitan cities also have private gymnastic clubs.

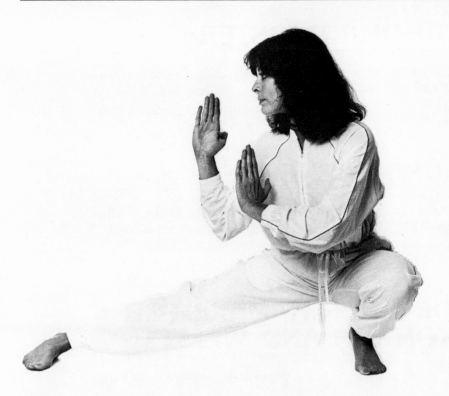

Karate. Properly practiced and supervised karate can be a safe and enjoyable pastime. Private exercise halls (called dojos) are quite common in all metropolitan areas and are becoming easier to find in small towns. Make sure the instructor is qualified, and you'll be on your way to boosting your stomach and waist reshaping, since the majority of the moves called for require power from your middle body muscles. Exaggerated low-stance work quickly shapes thighs, front, back, and side.

Jazz dancing. A type of dance you're likely to see on the Broadway stage. A vigorous way to condition the middle of your body. As you move to music, your body beautifies. You'll bend and stretch every which way, and all those high kicks will build terrific stomach muscles and beautifully sculptured thighs. Check the Yellow Pages under Dance Instruction for classes in your locality.

AT-HOME BOOSTERS

Unfortunately there isn't much in your daily routine that can be used to reduce your waist and stomach, which is probably why that area got out of shape in the first place.

FRINGE BENEFITS

As you reshape your stomach, waist, and front thighs, you'll be pleased to note response from your chin and neck areas. Slack necks pick up a bit and double chins fall by the wayside.

TORTURE CHAMBER FOR STOMACH AND WAIST

Do either of these exercises, or alternate them from day to day for variety.

Leg Raises
Repetition goal: one hundred leg raises.

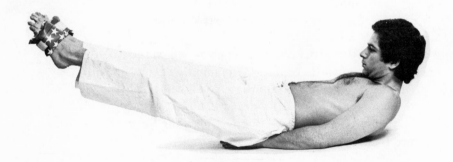

Do your leg raises exactly as described earlier in this chapter. The only difference is where you wear your body weights. Put them around your insteps. Moving the weight from your ankle to your foot exerts a much bigger pull on the middle body muscles and is, therefore, more difficult.

Flutters

Repetition goal: two hundred flutters (that's one hundred on each leg).

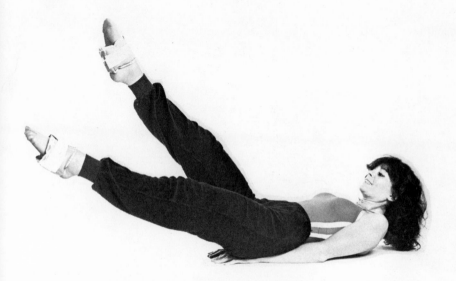

Again, do this exercise exactly as directed earlier in this chapter. Just change the position of your body weights from your ankles to your instep.

Chapter 8

Inner Thigh, Inner Knee

My mailbox usually includes letters asking for inner leg toners. They are always fraught with frustration. "Everyone writes articles and teaches exercises for the outside of the leg, what about me and my inner lumps and bumps?" "The rest of my body is in great shape, I'm not overweight and yet I have ugly lumps of fat on the inside of my knees, help!" "I'm too embarrassed to put on a bathing suit this year, the skin is just hanging on the inside of my legs."

Your inner leg requires conditioning and care just like every other part of the body. The inside of the thighs and knees are very prone to flab. Deposits of fat on the inner thigh and knee are an indication that circulation is poor in that area. Along with slack hanging skin, flab means that the muscles underneath are crying for attention. Both problems are probably due to the fact that you spend a lot of time sitting.

Inside thigh looseness is shared by men and women, and is the only upper leg problem that is. All the men I have queried who suffer from this have had jobs that require long hours of chair time.

You can cheer up because the inside of the thigh and the inside of the knee are relatively easy areas to zero in on and reshape. They both respond quickly to an all-out attack.

First, you must break bad habits that contribute to your inner leg problem. Be sure to concentrate on all aspects of your reshaping program during this "Magical Month."

Circulation constrictors will lead to the breakdown of free and easy blood flow and will contribute to fat deposits. Here are some do's and don'ts to keep in mind.

Don't cross your legs while sitting. This is a hard habit to break and the greatest contributor to ugly legs. Here's a trick to help you overcome the habit and make your back feel better at the same time: place a couple of books under your feet when you are sitting and make sure the back of your hips touch the back of your chair. This should set your knees a little higher than your hips. Now, put a pencil across your knees. Every time you go to cross your legs, the pencil will fall and remind you not to. I'm sure you will find this a much more comfortable work position. It is certainly a healthier one than most desk workers assume.

Don't wear girdles or support hose. Unless you are wearing a constricting device under doctor's orders, forget about those circulation hamperers. They quickly lead to muscle slackness and fat deposits.

If your problem is hard fat, *you must massage* it during this period to help break it down. The inner knee sometimes holds the hardest lumps of fat on the body: use a natural bristle brush or a loofah. Make circles with your massage tool over the area that is holding lumps. Continue to make circles until the skin becomes rosy and you can feel strong circulation there. Go easy at first. This "dry massage" is extremely beneficial in the fight to bring free blood flow back to an area. When you are finished, you will see an ashlike grey dust on your skin. Those are dead skin cells you needed to be rid of so that your skin can breathe properly and begin to function again. Now take a shower or wash the area you massaged. Use the skin oil described in chapter thirteen as the finishing step. Be sure not to neglect this very important step. Your overall result will be much faster and more pleasing to the eye. This reshaping massage should be an everyday occurrence for you, and if you like the feeling, try this dry massage on your entire body!

Don't consume large amounts of dairy products such as milk, cheese, and butter. If you can just forget the dairy for a month, you'll be pleased with the quick results.

If your problem is hanging skin, I would like you to add at least one nutritional skin toner to your diet (see chapter thirteen) and to use the body lotion recommended in chapter thirteen. Take your choice of these skin-feeding, tasty drinks: four ounces of carrot juice and four ounces of cucumber juice or four ounces of carrot juice mixed with four ounces of green pepper juice. Both of these eight-ounce servings must be freshly made and taken immediately. They cannot be stored, canned, or bottled. If you don't have a vegetable juicer, try your neighborhood juice bar. Drink a big glass or two every day! Make sure your diet is high in B-complex factors, so necessary to healthy skin. A vitamin supplement will solve that lack if you haven't time to seek them out in food form. (If you do, mung bean sprouts and alfalfa sprouts, eaten raw, would provide lots of skin nutrition for you.)

CHANGE YOUR WARM-UP

Do your regular count of jumping jacks or rope jumping. Increase your open-leg stretches to a count of fifty each.

As soon as you finish your warm-up do the open-and-close exercise.

Open-and-Close

You may start with less, and take a week to build to your full count, in small sets if necessary.

1. Put three-pound body weights on your ankles.
2. Lie on your back on the floor and lift your legs until they are at right angles to your body.
3. Open your legs until you feel a good pull on the inside of your thighs, then close them. Work very slowly. Repeat.

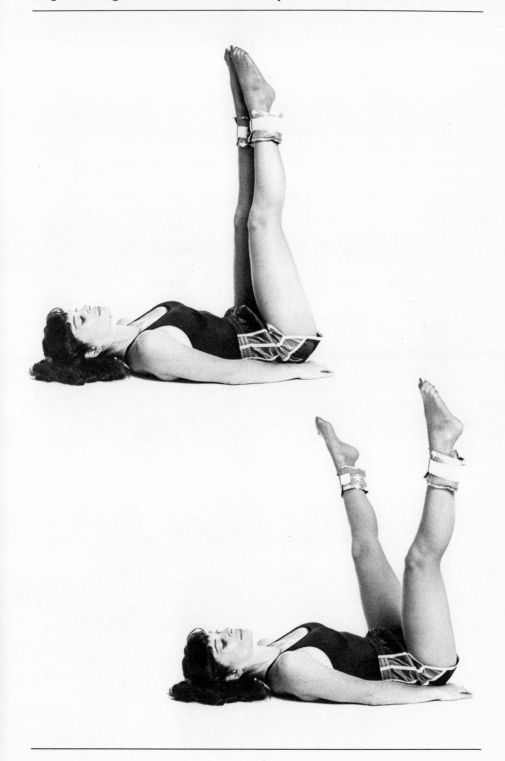

Repetition goal: one hundred a day.

Scissors

These scissors are interchangeable with the open-and-closes. You may do half of each on the same day, or scissors one day, open-and-closes the next.

1. Put three-pound body weights on your ankles.
2. Lie on your back on the floor and lift your legs until they are at right angles to your body.
3. Slowly open your legs until you feel a good pull on the inside.
4. Bring your legs together in a right-over, left-cross position.
5. Slowly open again.
6. Bring your legs together in a left-over, right-cross position.
7. Repeat, alternating right crosses and left crosses.

Make sure to finish your inner leg workout by going upside down. Most beneficial to you would be a Yogic shoulder stand or a Yogic plow position.

A double whammy for your inner legs is a shoulder stand accompanied by leg bicycles. If you can't get all the way up to your shoulders, make sure to rest your legs higher than your head for at least two full minutes after your workout.

Repetition goal: one hundred a day.

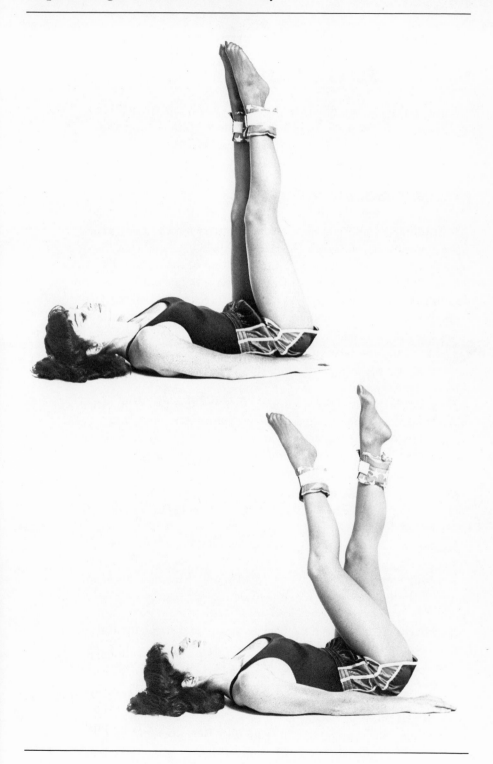

INNER THIGH AND INNER KNEE BOOSTERS

Since you've promised to conduct an all-out assault on the inside of your legs, I know you will pick one or more of these fun and home boosters to speed along your reshaping program.

Playtime Boosters

Swimming. Even if you don't know how to swim, you can do this water booster for your inner legs. *Use a flutterboard.* Hold it with your hands, and keep the front tip up and out of the water. (The board will hold your weight, so you don't have to be able to swim to do this marvelous-for-your-legs workout.) Execute the froglike kick from the breast stroke. Push that board back and forth through the water for at least fifteen nonstop minutes. A half hour is the goal for you to work up to. Remember, while you're working out, the water is giving you a massage. This double attack on the inner leg is a miracle worker.

Bicycle. Here's your chance to help the pollution problem, conserve energy, save money, and shape up your inner thighs and knees. Plain bike or fancy ten speed, whatever your pleasure, will work wonders for your legs. Spend at least an hour biking nonstop; and remember, the more hills you go up the better the workout.

Dancing. A musical, social solution to your inner leg problem. Disco will give you the best workout with a partner. For solo dance, try jazz class or ballet.

Jogging will help you reshape. Do at least a mile, three times a week.

Jumping rope is great for inner legs. Do it to disco music, use a wide variation of steps. An LP runs fifteen to eighteen minutes — all the time you need to jump into super shape.

Backpacking and hiking. Go back to nature and shape up at the same time.

Cross-country skiing. Often called Nordic skiing, this national sport of Scandinavian countries is rapidly becoming a popular recreational pastime in America. The intensity of your skiing is variable; the terrain, your pace, and the length of your rest periods determine how hard a workout you're getting. But, whether you push or take it easy, your inner legs will shape up.

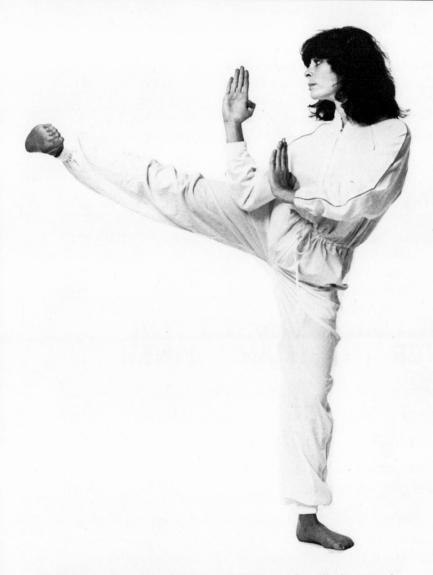

Martial arts. Kung Fu, karate, and Taikwondo will give you the best leg workouts. Killer stances will shape your inner thighs and knees. High kicking will shape up your entire lower body.

At-home Boosters

Stair climbing is extremely effective as an inner leg shaper. At work or at home, you can find all kinds of excuses to climb stairs. If you have stairs at home, you can climb up and down them to music. As your legs get stronger, take two, then three steps at a time. Try to build to fifteen minutes of nonstop stair climbing.

FRINGE BENEFITS

As you tone and reshape your inner legs, your stomach will receive some benefit.

TORTURE CHAMBER FOR INNER THIGH AND INNER KNEE

You asked for it!

Leg Scissors and Leg Open-and-Closes
Repetition goal: one hundred.

You may alternate between the two exercises, but, this time, *add weight*. You'll need two pairs of three-pound body weights for this particular torture. Wear one pair on your ankles and one pair on your insteps. That's a total of six pounds on each leg.

Do the exercises exactly as described earlier in this chapter.

WATER TORTURE

If you have access to a swimming pool, you can substitute a workout on the flutterboard for 45 minutes for the above exercises.

NOT TO WORRY

Inner thighs and inner knees may seem to lump up at the beginning of your reshaping exercises. Don't get excited, just keep working. Your legs are going to go through a few different phases before they smooth out to perfection. Remember, your legs have been neglected for a long while, so have patience with your body as it pulls slack muscles together.

Chapter 9

Outside of the Upper Hip and Thighs

Well, here we go full blast into almost every woman's figure failure. The nicknames for this susceptible-to-fat area are imaginative: thigh bulge, saddlebags, riding breeches . . . the names may be cute but the sight isn't. And how the bearers of these appendages hate them! It is impossible to appear attractive in jeans, shorts, bathing suits, straight-lined skirts — the list goes on and on.

Plastic surgeons have an operation specifically for this area. The procedure is painful, leaves large scars, and is extremely expensive. The worst of it is that the ugly lumps return shortly after the medical trauma if the patient doesn't change her eating or exercise habits. Don't even consider this nonsolution to your problem!

Why do so many women have this problem in common? First of all, women naturally have more fat on their bodies than men. (This is a survival advantage — women take longer to starve to death than men.) One of the first places for additional fat to build up is on the thighs. Because of low circulation and lack of muscle tone in that area, you can expect even the smallest amount of extra poundage to locate there. If your system were flowing properly, fat would be more evenly distributed on your body. Now, how did you manage to accumulate extra fat? What's stopping up your system?

Your problem is half physical, half nutritional. This outside hip and thigh problem plagued Ellen also. She attacked it from every angle, you should too.

You have your side body bulges partly because you ate them on. Certain foods can be major contributors to hard-packed fat and bad circulation. Dr. Paavo Airola, author of ten books on diet and nutrition, says to watch out for dairy foods (milk, cheese, butter), chemicals (food additives and preservatives), beef and pork, salt, all forms of sugar (alcohol, white bread, white rice, pasta, and refined cereals are all sugars once ingested).

If you are more than ten pounds overweight, you must go on a diet in order to smooth out this area. If you're not overweight, but are holding hard-packed fat on your thighs, try to eliminate meat and dairy products from your diet during the "Magical Month." Substitute raw fruits and vegetables. Melons are "living food," chock full of enzymes to help your circulation move. Make sprout salads an everyday occurrence. Make and drink a body flusher (see chapter twelve).

You must massage the outside of your legs and hips every day during the "Magical Month." It won't take you long, but it's an important part of your reshaping program. Details for massaging hard fat are outlined in chapter thirteen.

I'm going to shoot straight from the shoulder here. This is the hardest area on the body to reshape. Ellen says she thought it would never give. You will do it — and within the allotted time period. But you are going to have to work hard and *have patience,* because this area will not respond until what seems like the bitter end. Many people get discouraged and begin to question the program, but, if you stick it out, suddenly your whole problem area will smooth out. So, please trust me, and stay with it.

I want you to give your circulation every chance to flow through this area. Here are a couple of rules that will make you feel good and will speed you along your toning: don't wear girdles, don't wear support hose. Both these upper-body constrictors are harmful to your health and shape. Don't cross your legs while sitting. If you have a desk job, place a book or two under your feet. This will set your knees higher than your hips. Make sure the back of your hips touch the back of the chair. This correct sitting posture relieves pressures on your lower back. Now, place a pencil across your knees. Every time you return to your harmful leg-crossing habit, the pencil will hit the floor and remind you.

If you are dieting, remember that your body drops weight from the top down. So don't get discouraged if bulges don't seem to be responding to your diet. They will — just have patience and, rest assured, the outsides of the upper hip and, particularly, the thigh will be the very last locations on your body to drop fat.

If you seem to be bulking up, try to ride the period through. What's actually happening is that your muscle is responding to the exercise, making the overlying fat appear bigger. This look will alter as you build the muscle to the point where it will contour the outside of the leg. If, at the end of the "Magical Month," your whole upper thigh measures larger than before but looks much better, you are ahead of the game. Remember, you're working for appearance, not numbers.

Since we are all different, you may be a rare exception. If you feel that you are bulking excessively, counter it by swimming. Don't stop the exercise under any circumstances, just add the water exercise. If you can't swim, you must then do extra stretching, particularly open-leg stretches. Double your count to hold the stretch and do this leg elongator several times a day.

Pay strict attention to the form involved in the following exercise. Don't be haphazard, or your outside hip and thigh will appear the same.

As soon as you finish your warm-up do side leg raises.

Side Leg Raises

You may start with less, but quickly advance to your full count.

1. Attach three-pound body weights to your ankles.
2. Lie on your side. Position your top body for comfort. It may be touching the floor or be supported by your arms. Time and practice will determine your own preference. But, you must tip your hip down toward the floor. Make sure your navel points at the floor.
3. Very slowly raise your top leg as high as you can.
4. Slowly, slowly, lower the leg behind your body to one inch from the floor. Do not touch the floor!
5. After you've completed the count on one side, turn on your other side and repeat the exercise with your other leg. If you touch the floor between raises you will remove tension from the area you need to work on. It is extremely important, when working on this outside hip and thigh, that you *lift*, not throw, your weight upward. Your upper body should not move at all!

Finish your outside leg workout by going upside down. Do a shoulder stand and move your legs in a bicycle motion for a minute or two, then just rest in a plow or shoulder stand. If you are not familiar with these Yogic stands, do be sure to place your feet higher than your head for at least two minutes.

Repetition goal: one hundred on each leg.

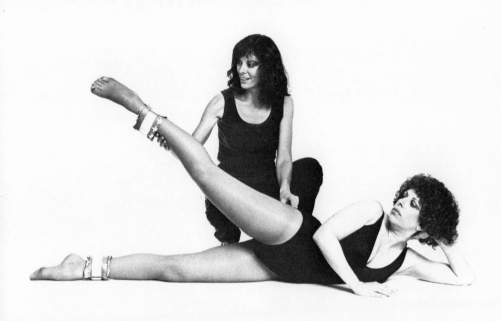

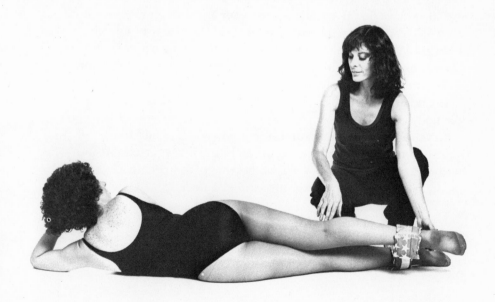

OUTSIDE HIP AND THIGH BOOSTERS

Playtime Boosters

Be sure to pick one of these boosters and reap the benefits!

Jump rope. For melting down a bulky upper hip, nothing is faster. Fifteen minutes a day is an adequate time period. Use a variation of steps, and do your rope jumping to disco music. Your thighs will respond best to a three-time-a-week rope-skipping schedule.

Jogging. A perfect exercise for upper hip and thigh. The heel-toe action is just what you need to shake up the spots you're working on. I find alternating between jogging and jumping rope also very successful for hitting this area.

Swimming. Even if you don't know how to swim, you can do this water booster for your outside thighs and hips. *Use a flutterboard.* Hold it with your hands and keep the front tip up and out of the water. (The board will hold your weight, so you don't have to be able to swim to do this marvelous-for-your-legs workout.) Execute the froglike kick from the breast stroke and the flutter kick from the crawl. Alternate the two kicks between laps. One lap of frog kicking, one lap of flutter kicking. Work up to a nonstop half hour every time you take to the water. (Ellen worked up to a full hour on the flutterboard, when she realized how beautifying to her bottom body it was.)

Bicycling. A good shape-up for your outside hips and thighs. But, you must put on the speed. Go up hills. Push yourself. Meandering along at a relaxed pace is no good. Try to work up a sweat. Spend at least an hour biking, three times a week.

Karate. The low sweeps and stances, the high kicks, and the forced-pace workout will shape up your hips and thighs very quickly. Make sure you find a school that works hard. USA GoJu, Chinese GoJu, and Taikwondo are some systems of karate that are known for their classic workouts. (Ellen worked at martial arts once a week during her reshape.)

Racquet sports will have you running after the ball and working your upper hips and thighs like crazy. Tennis, racquet ball, and squash are all effective boosters.

Gymnastics. Free exercise is your best bet.

Ballet. The discipline of the bar will pull your outer lines into shape. Take three classes a week. Seek out a strict and classical school. Your posture will improve along with your body outline.

Jazz dance. A la Ann Margret. For a nonstop body shaper, you can't beat moving to jazz rhythm. Make sure it's a fast moving class. Take a look at the instructor's body. If it's lean and hard, that's a good class for you.

Roller skating. The newest movement craze to hit America. Roller rinks are opening everywhere and the beat is disco. The parks are filled with skaters on special teflon wheels to handle concrete. Join them. Skate for hours: it's fun and a wonderful hip and thigh shaper.

Fencing. The beautiful lunging movements of this sport are wonderful upper leg and hip shapers.

Handball. A super-fast-moving sport that will have your legs and hips shaped up in no time.

At-home Boosters

Wash dishes in a "horse" stance. With both toes pointing forward and shoulder-width apart, assume a semisquat position. Try not to let your feet splay out too widely and keep your knees wide open. You will immediately feel the tension on your thighs. This "horse" stance is a killer and a karate basic. It was originally developed by ancient Chinese martial artists who sought to develop stability on moving boats.

Keep your back straight. Use this stance whenever you have a standing job to do. Even brushing your teeth can contribute to your reshaping if you do it in a "horse." (I am in a "horse" as I type this chapter. My version of killing two birds with one stone.)

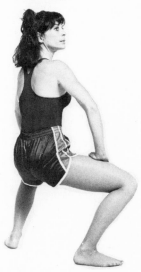

Stair climbing. Don't use elevators. The higher the floor, the better for your problem area. Think of excuses to go up and down stairs. As you get used to climbing, take them two and even three steps at a time. This will give you stretch and work at the same time.

FRINGE BENEFITS

The side leg raises will affect the waist (at the side) and be of some benefit to the buttocks and back of the thighs.

TORTURE CHAMBER FOR OUTER HIP AND THIGH

Side Leg Raises
Repetition goal: one hundred lifts on each leg.

Do your leg raises exactly as described earlier in this chapter, but wear two body weights on each leg: one three-pound weight on your ankle, and one three-pound weight on your instep.

Now you are working with six pounds. Be sure to lift, not throw, the weight up, and bring your leg down slowly.

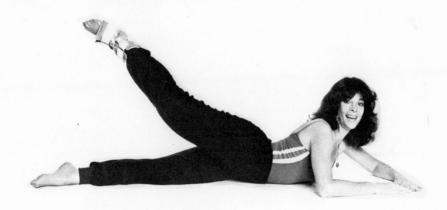

NOT TO WORRY

Of all the areas on the body to reshape, the outside hip and thigh are the scariest to wait out. As the lax muscles respond to hard work, the area between the hip and upper thigh pulls in. This makes the upper hip and thigh appear larger and bulkier. At this point in their reshaping program, exercisers send panic-stricken letters: "Everything looks worse, I'm ruined." And they even send accompanying sketches to demonstrate their lament.

This unsightly period can last from two days to two weeks. Ride it out! It will get better. Don't stop working at this point. Rather, take it as encouragement. The in-and-out shape your outer hip and thigh has temporarily taken on is a positive sign. It means your muscles are working and responding as expected. Stay with it!

Chapter 10

Buttocks and Back Thigh

What could be more discouraging than possessing a hanging behind in this age of designer jeans? Droopy buttocks are impossible to hide in pants — or shorts. Bathing suits really reveal the back-view problem.

The buttocks are nature's fat cupboards, and if you've extra on your body, you can bet a good portion of it is there. The muscles in your buttocks are large. When they are not properly conditioned, the rear end appears flat and long instead of rounded and high. Luckily, the buttocks respond quickly to the reshaping exercise I'm going to give you.

The back of the thigh can be a nestling place for hard fat. In that space just under the buttocks, ridges, lumps, and bumps abound. You can fix up the eyesore by smoothing out the area. Or the back of the leg can appear flat, with no shape. That can be corrected also. As soon as you pump up the muscle, a rounded well-sculptured upper leg emerges.

We will be working on the area from the back of your waist down to the back of your knees. When you are finished with the "Magical Month," you will have a smooth well-rounded backside that will look good in a pair of jeans.

Most people who want to reshape their backsides have a dual problem: they are overweight and have lost muscle tone. If this description fits you, understand that you will not necessarily reduce the size of your rear, but that it will have a better shape. The exercises may reduce the girth of your buttocks at the lower portion but make it bigger at the top. This is the result of the muscle responding and picking up hanging fat. If you want to reduce your buttocks while reshaping them, you must go on a diet if you're more than ten pounds overweight.

I want you to use strong massage on your buttocks and thighs. You will find directions in chapter thirteen. Remember, we're going to hit this area with everything at once, that's the secret to reshaping.

Why are the muscles slack in your buttocks and back thighs? Because of nonuse and restriction of circulation. You are definitely going to use your muscles and bring them back to shape this month, so in order to get strong circulation flowing again, watch out for these circulation constrictors:

If you sit long hours, *be sure not to cross your legs.* Here's a health hint to improve your posture, prevent back pain, and break a leg-crossing habit. Put a phone book under your feet while you sit. This should raise your knees above your hips. Make sure the back of your hips are against the back of your chair. Place a pencil across your legs. It will hit the floor if you try to cross them. Now that you've raised the level of your legs, they won't press against the chair edge anymore. Your circulation will not be inhibited for many hours each day.

If you're sitting hours are spent driving a car, position your car seat so that your knees are higher than your hips.

Don't wear girdles or support hose. Both are health hazards. They restrict your circulation.

Double up on the open-leg stretching in your warm-up by holding the count for fifty. Do four of these stretches. You will feel the pull on the muscles in your buttocks and back of your thighs as you stretch. That's good and will also aid your circulation.

As soon as you finish your warm-up, do both of the following exercises.

Bent Leg Pushes

You may start with less, but hurry to your goal.

1. Wear three-pound weights on your ankles.
2. Lie flat on your stomach, or you may support your upper body with your arms, whichever is more comfortable for you.
3. Bend your leg at the knee and push your heel skyward.
4. Bring the knee down to an inch from the floor and push back upward. *Do not touch the floor between pushes,* or you will take tension off your muscles and defeat your purpose.

Half Leg Lifts

You may start with less, but this is an easy exercise and you should meet your goal quickly.

1. Keep your leg weights on. Lie flat on your stomach, or you may support your upper body with your arms.
2. Bend your leg at the knee.
3. Lower it back down to one inch from the floor.
4. Repeat.

Do not touch the floor between lifts!

If you place your fingers on the back of your thigh as you do this exercise, you will feel the muscle responding. Try to keep your fingers there for a while and feel how you can keep the most tension on those muscles as you work.

I usually alternate bent leg pushes and half leg lifts to make rear body workouts more interesting. Do a set of one, then a set of the other. If your muscle response is fast and you like what's happening, I would suggest moving into the "Torture Chamber" after you become accustomed to the amount of weight you are working with. These are big muscles and you can really push them along.

Repetition goal: one hundred bent leg pushes on each leg.

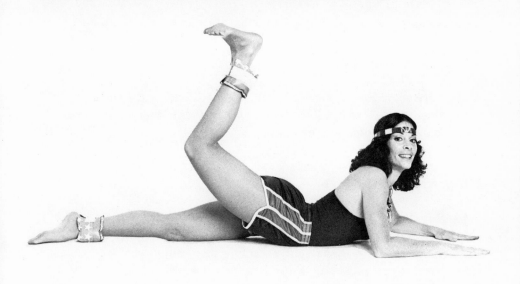

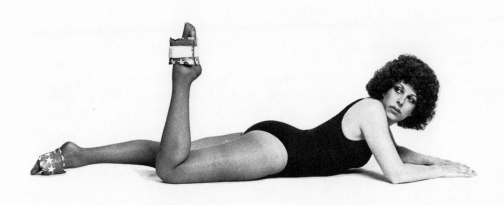

Repetition goal: fifty half leg lifts on each leg.

BUTTOCKS AND BACK THIGH BOOSTERS

Here are your choices. Pick one that appeals to you, or try them all. Indulge as often as possible. Remember, this is another way to speed along your reshaping program.

Playtime Boosters

Jogging. Join the craze. Nothing will boost your buttock and back thigh reshaping quite as fast as the heel-toe action required for jogging. Be sure to wear a good running shoe, with a wide spread heel so that maximum shock is absorbed while you run. If you're not tuned in to jogging yet, you may start with a walk, jog, walk program until you build up your stamina a bit. If you don't want to get involved with crowds of runners, you can jog around your house, outside or inside. Just be sure to find out the distance you are covering, and do at least one mile each time you jog. If you are doing walk, jog, walk, do at least two miles.

Swimming. Grab a flutterboard, keep the front tip out of the water, and hold the board with both hands. Push the flutterboard through the water with your legs. Use the froglike kick to the breast stroke and the flutter kick that usually accompanies the crawl. Alternate between the two kicks for a full half hour. This is easy to do even if you can't swim, as the board holds you up and just your legs are moving. This is a surefire way to shape up buttocks and back thighs. The water is massaging you all the time you're working your muscles. The double benefit will show up as firm rounded contours.

Jumping rope may be alternated with jogging. Since you're on your toes all the time you skip rope, your body receives different benefits than those derived from the heel-toe action of jogging. Take advantage of both for your reshaping.

Hiking. Go out to the countryside for fresh air and a shape-up. Both the up and down climbing you'll do on the trail will use just the area of your body you want to reshape.

Bicycling. You can use a stationary indoor type, or head for the bike paths outside. Your upper legs and rear will respond to the pushing movement necessary to turn your pedals. Indoor stationary bikes can be set for resistance, but it takes an hour of outdoor biking to make a difference. Don't make it easy on yourself. The more difficulty in the exercise, the better the result.

Disco dancing. Hours of dancing are wonderful for your problem area. The faster the beat, the more of a workout you'll receive. Refresh yourself with white wine spritzers instead of drinking hard liquor while you're out on the town. Or best of all, pass up the alcohol and just indulge in dance.

Karate. High kicks, low stances, and sweeps will shape up your entire bottom body in record time! Make sure it's a hard-working class, look for USA GoJu, karate, or Taikwondo.

Dance class. Jazz and ballet will lead to a beautiful bottom body. Both disciplines call on your lower muscles to push and stretch and leap.

Gymnastics. A rewarding experience for your body. The free exercise is for you. Try your local Y or the Yellow Pages for a private club.

At-home Boosters

Open leg stretching. It's a good idea to sit around in this open leg stretch. TV watching can aid your buttock and thigh reduction. Just sit on the floor and stretch as you take in your favorite program.

Stair climbing will shape your thighs and buttocks. Find excuses to go up and down stairs. You're doing yourself a big favor. Forget about elevators during the "Magical Month."

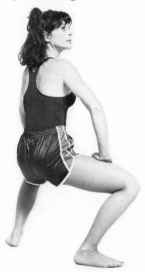

Use **the "horse" stance** for washing dishes, brushing your teeth, or any standing task. Point both your feet forward and drop your seat toward the ground. This karate power stance is a terrific bottom-body shaper.

FRINGE BENEFITS

The bent leg pushes will help to smooth out a side thigh bulge. For a really perfect upper leg, one should exercise front, side, and back. Add the front leg raises (see pp. 90–91) and side leg raises (see pp. 116–117) to the bent leg pushes.

TORTURE CHAMBER FOR BUTTOCKS AND BACK THIGH

Do both these exercises just as they were described earlier in this chapter, but wear two sets of body weights: one three-pound weight on your ankle and another three-pound weight on your instep for a total of six pounds on each leg.

Bent Leg Pushes
Repetition goal: one hundred on each leg.

Half Leg Lifts
Repetition goal: fifty on each leg.

For the best workout, alternate between the two exercises. Do a set of one, then a set of the other. You're working with six pounds of weight now and you may feel some muscle soreness. That's okay. Push ahead.

Chapter 11

Calves and Ankles

The phrase, a "well-turned ankle," encompasses the entire lower leg. It's unlikely that the compliment would be made were the ankle attached to a bulging or withered calf. So, we are going to reshape your leg from the knee down to fit that flattering maxim.

I'm directing these calf and ankle reshaping exercises to women since I have yet to have a male ask for either. There are two different calf and ankle reshapings: one for overdeveloped lower legs and one for underdeveloped calves and ankles. Pick your category, and let's get started.

UNDERDEVELOPED CALVES AND ANKLES

Many women are interested in adding to their lower legs — making them bigger *and curvier*. It is not uncommon to see an otherwise attractive body appear out of balance and weak because of skinny, shapeless calves.

The function of the muscle located at the back of the calf is mainly to lift your heel from the floor. Without it, you wouldn't be able to walk. To see the calf muscle in action, stand sideways in a full-length mirror: rise up on your toes — watch the calf muscle bulge as it shortens, and then lengthen as you lower back downwards.

Many women have shortened, locked calf muscles and sore ankles from years of wearing high heels. If this has happened to you, it will be remedied by the exercises you use in your reshaping program.

Why is your calf muscle so flat and flaccid? Because if you wear high heels, you haven't called on it to fulfill its proper function in a long time: the heels have prevented the muscle from being stretched to its full length. If you haven't been involved in any active sports, your lower leg is probably out of shape. Sport enthusiasts develop their calves when they run, climb, and jump.

You may expect some pain from your reshaping exercises. As the shortened muscle stretches, and it must in order to look terrific, you will feel the years of nonuse. Just bear the discomfort, it's not serious, nor will it cause permanent damage. You can rest assured your reward will be a much more attractively shaped leg.

Pay special attention to your warm-up. Do your full count of one hundred jumping jacks or jump-rope skips. Double up on the count for your standing stretch. That's four stretches. Hold each one for the count of twenty-five. Don't skip your open leg stretch. This increased standing stretch is not a substitute, but an Achilles tendon stretcher to compensate for your shortened calf muscle and a must for your reshaping. As soon as you finish your warm-up do the following toe raises.

Toe Raises

1. Hold a three-pound body weight in each hand. Stand with both toes pointed forward. Spread your feet apart to your own shoulder width.
2. Rise up on your toes, raising your heels as far from the floor as possible, and hold a moment.
3. Slowly, lower your heels down *to one inch from the floor.*
4. Rise back up to your tiptoes.

Don't break the tension by touching your heels to the floor between raises.

When you finish your toe raises, do two more standing stretches. Hold each for the count of twenty-five.

Repetition goal: one hundred toe raises a day.

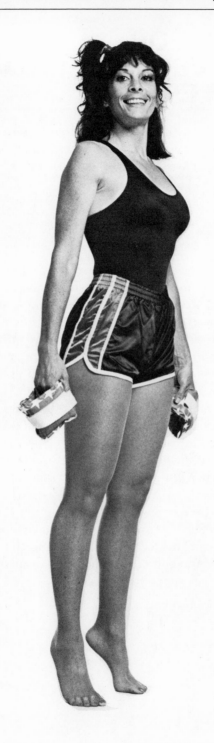

BOOSTERS FOR UNDERDEVELOPED CALVES AND ANKLES

Now is the time for you to indulge in sports that require mobility. Pick a booster that appeals to you and go at it steadily during the month of reshaping. Three times a week spent with any of these boosters will give you quick results.

Playtime Boosters

Jumping rope. This is the quickest way to shapely calves and ankles. Use a variety of steps, and do them to disco music. An album lasts fifteen to eighteen minutes — perfect jump-rope time for you. When the music is over, so is your workout. Be sure to wear proper athletic shoes and stay up on your toes all the time you're jumping. (For more information see chapter three.)

Ballet will keep you on your toes and leaping gracefully — just what your calves and ankles need for shaping.

Gymnastics. Free exercise, the floor work of gymnastics, requires you to take off into various moves filled with grace and mobility. Your calf muscles are called into play.

Basketball. Making for the hoop requires work by your calf muscles. Lots of leaping in this fast-paced team sport is just what you need for your shape-up.

Mountain climbing. Even in big cities there are intown mountain-climbing schools which take groups of students into local parks where they learn rock-climbing techniques for scaling high peaks. The workout is terrific. And best of all, your calves do all the pushing as you pretend you're conquering Everest.

At-home Boosters

Reach high. Do all the tasks you've been putting off that require standing on tiptoe. High shelves need rearranging, tops of closets can always use some attention. Look around, a lot of household chores require you to stretch. Substitute standing on tiptoe for stools or ladders.

Stand on tiptoe for dish washing, brushing teeth, waiting in a grocery market line — any standing time may be turned into a booster for your calves and ankles.

Climb stairs. Forget about elevators and escalators. If you live on a high floor, or work on one, make excuses to run up and down during the day. Your calves will love the exercise and shape up in appreciation.

Walk, don't ride, during this "Magical Month."

TORTURE CHAMBER FOR UNDERDEVELOPED CALVES AND ANKLES

You will feel your calf muscles singing to you after this killer. *Double up on standing stretches during your warm-up.* Do four stretches with a count of twenty-five for each.

Toe Raises on Book
Repetition goal: one hundred a day.

1. Stand with your toes on a fairly thick book. (Two inches is
   good.) Your heels should be on the floor. Keep your arms at
   your sides and hold a three-pound body weight in each hand.
2. Bring your heels as high as possible off the floor until you are
   on tiptoe on the book. Hold a moment and slowly, slowly, lower
   your heels back to the floor.

   Finish with two more standing stretches. Hold each for the count
of twenty-five. Feel the muscles in the back of your calves stretch.
Relax and breathe.

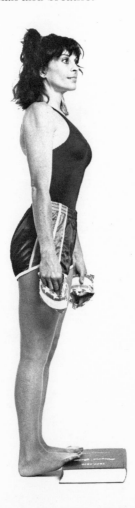 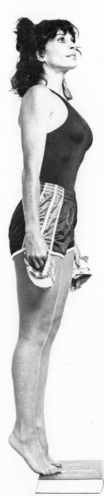

OVERDEVELOPED CALVES AND ANKLES

Swollen, puffy ankles are water holders; eliminating as much salt as possible from your diet will probably solve the problem. If you are not a salt user and your ankles swell, consult your doctor for causes and a solution.

Ankles and calves thickened with fat, particularly if the rest of your body is slim, respond very well to a concentrated, all-out assault. In addition to doing the exercises in this section, you should:

Control your diet. Reduce your intake of animal fat (dairy in particular) and make drinking a body flusher a daily habit. See chapter twelve for details.

Massage. Use daily intense deep massage as described in chapter thirteen.

Improve circulation by avoiding the wearing of girdles, support hose, and other circulation stoppers and by breaking yourself of the leg-crossing habit. Use this trick to do your back a favor and to allow blood to flow freely through your legs if you are in a sedentary occupation.

1. Place a telephone book (or two smaller books) under your feet at your desk. Make sure the back of your hips are against the back of the chair you are sitting in.
2. Place a pencil across your legs.

This will position your knees higher than your hips. Now the back of your knees won't press against the edge of the chair and cut off circulation. You will not feel so tired from sitting, and your grateful back will say, "thank you." If you start to cross your legs, the pencil will hit the floor and remind you to break this circulation-impairing habit.

Drivers should position car seats so their knees are pitched higher than their hips for the same reasons.

RESHAPERS FOR TOO-BIG CALVES AND ANKLES

If you've been wearing high heels for years, you may expect some calf pain as your shortened muscle stretches. The end result will be worth the discomfort. Your legs will feel better and look better with a properly elongated muscle. A bunched-up calf muscle appears bulky, a well-stretched calf muscle looks slim. Spend more time barefoot and add some low shoes to your wardrobe. Sandals are comfortable, and running shoes are all the rage now.

CHANGE YOUR WARM-UP

Do only fifty jumping jacks or rope jumps.

Increase your standing stretch. Do four and hold each stretch for the count of twenty-five.

Do both of the following exercises every day as soon as you finish your warm-up.

Heel and Toe Points

You should be able to hit this count very quickly. If you start with less, make sure you reach your goal within the first week of work.

1. Lie on the floor and stretch your arms out alongside your body.
2. Raise both legs all the way up to a right angle to your body.
3. Keep your legs still and point upward with your heels, then point upward with your toes.
4. Repeat.

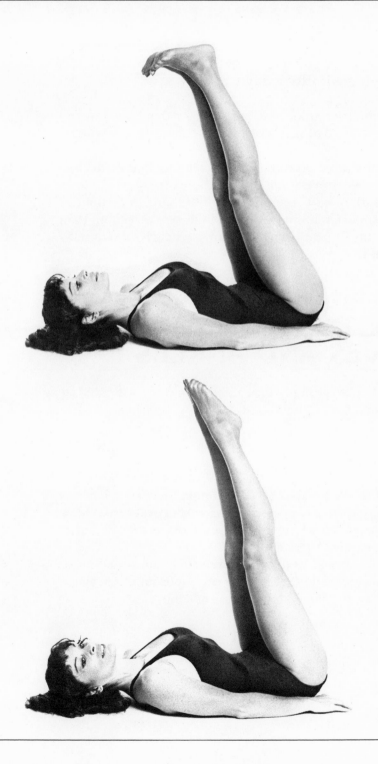

Foot Circles

Repetition goal: fifty a day.

This is another ankle and calf slimmer that should take you no time at all to reach your full goal.

1. Lie in the same position as for Heel and Toe Points and keep your legs very still during this exercise.
2. With both of your feet moving in the same direction, make small circles in the air. First in one direction, then in the other. Repeat twenty-five times in each direction, a total of fifty.

BOOSTERS FOR TOO-BIG CALVES AND ANKLES

Be sure to indulge in playtime and home activities to speed along your reshaping.

Playtime Boosters

Swim. The water is your best friend now. Circulation is what you need, and swimming is a top-drawer circulatory exercise. *The backstroke* is especially good for you. The crawl or freestyle is also a lower leg slimmer. Alternate your strokes.

Yoga. This ancient art of body movement requires you to spend a lot of time upside down. You'll get circulation and stretching work at the same time, with no muscle buildup.

At-home Boosters

Spend as much time as possible **upside down.** Watch TV with your legs higher than your head.

Knead, pinch, and **squeeze** your too-big calves and ankles. Besides your special massage (in chapter thirteen) grab a handful of lower leg while watching TV or just sitting. Push and pull, work the flesh, make the area red and flushed with circulation, then put your feet up higher than your head.

Try to sleep with your **feet and calves raised** with a pillow.

TORTURE CHAMBER FOR TOO-BIG CALVES AND ANKLES

Do your reshaping massage (see chapter thirteen for directions) twice each day. Morning and night will probably work best.

Take your choice or alternate between the two following tortures. Just make sure you indulge.

Swim for one half hour nonstop. Alternate between crawl and backstroke. *Use the flutterboard for ten minutes* of nonstop frog kicking (legs to the breast stroke). Grasp the flutterboard with your hands, keep the front tip out of the water and push with your legs. That's a total of forty minutes of water time.

Double up on both ankle and calf slimmers. That's one hundred heel and toe points and one hundred foot circles.

Chapter 12

Reshaping the Mostly Raw Food Way

You can speed along your reshaping this "Magical Month" by simply eating *whole meals* of either raw fruit or raw vegetables and grains instead of those containing meats, dairy products (milk, butter, cheese, cream), and nonnutritive foods such as sugar, white flour, and white rice. This allows you to eat as much food as you desire, while tremendously reducing the amount of calories you take in.

I know it isn't easy to change the food habits of a lifetime, but since you've decided to dedicate this month to improving your appearance — it's the perfect time to start.

Besides boosting your reshaping, raw foods, because they contain living enzymes and vitamins, will increase your energy, enhance the quality of your skin, and improve your general health. Another surprise benefit — drastically lowered food costs.

At the very least, you should add one of the following liquid and one solid body flusher to your diet each day. Try to substitute them for the equivalent items on your diet. Recipes for body flushers and directions for sprout growing may be found later in this chapter along with recipes for delicious whole raw meals. All liquids should be taken in eight-ounce sizes. Remember, take at least one liquid and one solid body flusher every day!

Liquids to Drop	*Body Flushing Substitutes*
Cow's milk	Half carrot, half celery juice
Coffee	Half carrot, half cucumber juice
Alcohol	Half carrot, half apple juice
Diet soda	Half carrot, half spinach juice
Soda	Watermelon juice (juice some rind
Canned, bottled, boxed juices	for a chyrophyll-rich drink)
	Cantaloupe juice
	Honeydew melon juice
	Rejuvelac
	Raisin rejuvelac

Solids to Drop	Body Flushing Substitutes
Meat	Sprout salads
Dairy from cows (cheese, milk, butter, cream)	Living cereal
	An entire meal of the melon of your choice.
White bread	
Pasta	
White rice	
Sugar	
Salt	
Refined cereals	

Don't bother with canned or bottled juices. Time and processing destroy their value. If you don't own a vegetable juicer, I strongly urge you to consider buying one. In the meantime, your neighborhood natural food store probably has a juice bar that will make your favorite juice to order.

Be sure to drink vegetable juices as soon as they are made. Never try to refrigerate juices, since the valuable vitamins dissipate in a short while.

I often order two juices for lunch. They are filling, low in calories, high in energy, delicious, and, according to Dr. Ann Wigmore, healing.*

Substituting fruit meals for meat meals. I believe in monofruit eating. That means having just one kind of fruit, and as much of it as you want per meal.† I often make a meal of honeydew melons, because besides being delicious, they contain the most enzymes of all the fruits. A body-flushing fruit meal will leave you feeling light and looking the same way.

Sprout salads as body flushers. Make them a whole meal or a side dish. Like the fruit meals, you can eat as much as your heart desires. You can buy alfalfa (the most healing of all the sprouts and the richest in chyrophyll), mung (a wonderful source of vitamin A), and soy (protein-rich sprout) in almost any store that carries fresh vegetables. But, it's cheaper and more fun to grow your own. I always have fresh wheat sprouts as they are particularly nutritious. In four days of sprouting, the vitamin E content of wheat increases

---

Make Your Juicer Your Drugstore (Wethersfield, Conn.: Omangod Press, 1978).
† For more information on monofruit eating, see Dr. Viktoras Kulvinskas's *Survival into the 21st Century* (Wethersfield, Conn.: Omangod Press, 1977).

300 percent and some of the vitamin B complex components increase from 20 to 600 percent! People ask, "Isn't wheat terribly fattening?" Yes. If it's not sprouted. The difference between a dormant seed and a sprouted seed is astounding. For instance, one pound of wheat contains one thousand four hundred and ninety-seven calories. One pound of *sprouted wheat* contains only three hundred calories. So don't worry, go ahead and eat all the sprouts you want. For more about the nutritional values of sprouts, see the reading list at the back of this book.

THE MOSTLY RAW FOOD DIET

If you're more than ten pounds overweight, you must go on a diet in order for your reshaping program to work. I recommend the mostly raw-food diet that was so successful for Ellen. It's an easy one to follow, with no calories to count and no rigid meal plan to adhere to. It is also the diet I live on and have for the last six years. I attribute my overabundance of energy to it, my steady body weight and my general good health. But, the main reason I enjoy living on this diet is that I like to eat. Now I don't count calories or limit my food intake — all I have to do is not eat certain foods and I can have as much as I want of the hundreds of choices available. The time I save in food preparation is extensive. Making raw-food meals is always quick and easy. One just makes meals from the raw vegetables or raw fruit that appeals at the moment. Simply walk into any fruit and vegetable store and pick out what looks good and fresh that day. If you go to business, it's really easy to take fruit along for lunch. Restaurants offer varieties of delicious raw vegetable salads. Japanese cuisine is perfect for you on this diet, and their restaurants offer wide selections of raw foods. If you find yourself in a restaurant for dinner and cannot order raw foods, stick with vegetable and fish dishes. Italian cooking is known for delightful vegetable dishes, and since this is a *mostly* raw-food diet, you won't do yourself any harm by having a cooked meal now and then.

It is conceivable that a too-sudden switch to a raw-food regime after years of existing on a diet of refined and cooked foods could give you some digestive discomfort. So ease into it slowly and check with your doctor or nutritionist.

I've given you two weeks of taste-tempting recipes and snacks that go along with the diet. Once you get into the swing of raw-food things, your imagination will lead you to many more delicious dishes. First, here's how to grow sprouts for salads and cereals, and make rejuvelacs.

SPROUTS, REJUVELACS, AND LIVING CEREAL

Buy a large mason jar. Remove the inner disk from the lid and replace it with copper screen, plastic window mesh, nylon, or cheesecloth — whatever is easiest and handiest for you. Just a piece of cheesecloth, held on with a rubber band, is fine. If you want to get fancy, sprouting jars with permanent screens are available in natural food stores.

Rinse your seeds thoroughly and soak them overnight, with at least two parts water to one part seeds. Use water of a tepid temperature. (I use bottled spring water.) The smaller the seed, the less soaking time needed. Alfalfa will do with only three hours, but won't be harmed by up to fifteen. Larger seeds, such as chickpea, soy, and mung, may be soaked up to twenty hours.

In the morning, after the initial soaking, turn your jar upside down and pour off the water into a container (and save for rejuvelac). The mesh will allow the water to go, the seeds to remain.

Without removing the mesh, rinse the seeds and pour off the water again. Now place the jar in a dark place (I use my cupboards) upside down and slightly tipped, so that air can enter.

Rinse twice a day.

On the third day, place your sprouts in the window with the jar tipped so air enters. The sun will turn them green with healthy chlorophyll. The sprouts are ready to eat after one day's exposure to sun.

Buy your seeds at a natural food store. Good seeds for sprouting are wheat, alfalfa, mung, and soy bean. Sunflower seeds are spicy. Mung are nutlike, wheat are sweet. You'll have to experiment and find your favorites.

Rejuvelacs

Rejuvelac is the soak water from seeds. It is teeming with water-soluble nutrients and enzymes, and may be used as a drink by itself. It has a wheylike taste as a result of the living lactobacilli and yeasts. If the taste is too strong, you may cut the rejuvelac with spring water. Half and half makes a refreshing drink. Here are some rejuvelac flavor drinks.

Raisin Rejuvelac

Simply add a few raisins to your soaking seeds. The resulting rejuvelac is delicious and may be drunk as is or cut with spring water.

Fruit Rejuvelac

Use half rejuvelac and half or quarter freshly squeezed fruit juice. A bit of honey may be added for sweetener with lemon juice for a tasty lemonade.

I keep a supply of rejuvelacs in my icebox and they are always winners with guests. Children love rejuvelacs.

Other uses for rejuvelac are extensive. It can be used in sauces, soups, and for seed milk.*

Living Cereal

Soak wheat seeds for twelve to sixteen hours. Now the seeds are alive. Pour off the soak water and save for rejuvelac.

Serve the crunchy seeds with strawberries, blueberries, orange slices, bananas, or as the filling for a scooped-out melon. This is a first-class breakfast, loaded with vitamins, and so low in calories you can eat all you want.

Living cereal may be added to salads, eaten alone as a snack, or if ground, shaped into a patty and allowed to dry in the sun — as you would to make bread. Experiment with different seeds and see which taste you like best for your living cereal.

---

* Additional rejuvelac recipes may be found in Viktoras Kulvinskas's *Survival into the 21st Century* (Wethersfield, Conn.: Omangod Press 1977)

A MOSTLY RAW FOOD DAY

Breakfast (*choice of one*)
One kind of fruit
Living cereal
Living cereal and fruit

Lunch (*choice of one*)
Salad of your choice
One kind of fruit
Vegetable juice
Lunch crunch. (Mix living cereal with goat's milk yogurt, which may be purchased at a natural food store.)
An appetizer from the following recipe section.

Main Meal
Choose an appetizer and a main meal from the recipes that follow. Desserts are optional.

MOSTLY RAW RECIPES

Appetizers

Steamed Artichokes
(*One per person*)

Cut points off top of artichokes and stem off bottom. Stuff each artichoke with plenty of garlic pieces. Place in pot of low water (about one inch). Pour one tablespoon of olive oil over each artichoke. Cover and steam until you can pull any leaf out easily. (Usually about 15 to 20 minutes.) Serve as is. No sauce is needed, as the garlic and oil have made a delicious dressing while the artichoke steamed.

Stuffed Peppers

(*Serves two*)

Scoop out the green peppers so that you're left with a shell cup. Blend all other ingredients together by chopping or blending, and stuff the pepper shells with mixture.

2 green peppers
1 avocado
1/4 cup sprouts (mung are the spiciest)
1 tablespoon kelp (may be purchased in natural food store)
juice of 1/2 lemon
1/2 onion

Borscht

(*Serves two*)

Liquefy to desired consistency. May be served as soup or over sprouts salads as a delicious surprise dressing.

2 cups chopped beets
1/2 cup almonds
1 small green onion
2 cups rejuvelac (or beet juice or carrot juice or water)
1/2 lemon

Mushroom Stuffed with Green Garlic

(*Serves four*)

This dish may be prepared the day before eating, as it improves when left overnight.

Remove stalks from mushrooms and set aside the caps. In a bowl, squeeze garlic (or chop very fine). Chop the vegetables (you can use scissors) and add them to the garlic. Add the rest of the ingredients, check seasoning, then stuff the mixture into the mushroom caps. Place mushrooms upside down, on a plate. Refrigerate until ready to serve. The liquid in the mixture will be absorbed by the mushrooms, enhancing their flavor.

1 pound large mushrooms
2 cloves garlic
1 tablespoon spinach leaves
1 tablespoon chopped parsley
1 tablespoon watercress
1 teaspoon chives
1 teaspoon Dijon mustard
2 tablespoons apple cider vinegar
1/2 to 3/4 cup olive oil
sea salt
black pepper, freshly ground

Guacamole

(*Serves two*)

Use a fork and blend avocado to a creamy consistency, leaving a few lumps for texture. Mix with lemon and seasoning to taste. Add remaining ingredients. If you like spice, add freshly minced chili pepper or juice from crushed garlic.

1 avocado, diced
2 sweet red peppers, finely diced
2 tomatoes, diced
1 teaspoon kelp
1 lemon

Marinated Zucchini Slices

(*Serves four*)

Mix all ingredients together. Place in refrigerator to marinate for at least half an hour.

4 small zucchini, thinly sliced
juice from one lemon
3 tablespoons olive oil (raw)
1 clove crushed garlic
freshly ground black pepper

Green Pea Soup

(*Serves two*)

Whirl all ingredients in blender until creamy and smooth. If soup is too thick, thin with a little water or rejuvelac.

1 small avocado, peeled and
  chopped
1 cup green peas (fresh, of
  course)
1 tablespoon minced green onion
2 sprigs parsley or sweet basil
1 tablespoon lemon juice or 4
  cherry tomatoes

Marinated Asparagus

(*Serves two to three*)

Discard tough ends of asparagus. Chop stalks into bite-size pieces. Combine soy sauce, oil, and honey. Pour marinade over asparagus. Mix well and serve on a bed of sprouts.

1 pound asparagus
1 tablespoon soy sauce
1 tablespoon cold pressed sesame
  oil
2 teaspoons honey
alfalfa and mung bean sprouts

Stuffed Tomatoes with Avocado

(*Serves four*)

Hollow out a cavity in each tomato. Use a small amount of sea salt to salt the cavity. Chop avocado and insides of tomatoes and mix with other ingredients. Fill the tomato shells with this mixture. Sprinkle cayenne pepper on top and decorate with parsley.

2 avocados
juice of 2 lemons
4 large, firm tomatoes
1 cup mayonnaise (nondairy
  type, available at natural food
  stores)
1 teaspoon cayenne pepper
1 teaspoon fresh parsley, chopped
sea salt
black pepper, freshly ground
2 teaspoons fresh dill, chopped

Vichyssoise Verde

(Serves two)

Use two or more varieties of greens that are in season. Swiss chard and spinach, beet tops and celery, and lettuce and celery are tasty combinations.

Pour water into your blender. Add greens slowly, a little at a time. Reduce to a fine consistency. Add more greens if sauce is very thin. Blend in one optional ingredient to taste. Blend in avocado. Makes three cups.

2 cups greens (see below)
1/2 avocado
1 cup water or rejuvelac
1 teaspoon kelp
choose one: 3 mint leaves, 1/2
clove of garlic
3 scallion leaves
juice of one lemon,
one small onion

MAIN MEAL DISHES

Celery Nut Loaf with Sauce

(Serves four)

Mix all ingredients thoroughly in a bowl. Shape into a loaf. Put all ingredients for the sauce in blender, blend well, and top the nut loaf.

2 cups celery
1 cup raw almonds, ground
1 avocado, mashed
3 tablespoons onion, minced
3 tablespoons parsley, minced
1/2 teaspoon sage or thyme
juice of one small lemon
2 tablespoons mayonnaise

Sauce:
4 tomatoes
juice of one lemon
1 teaspoon honey
1/2 teaspoon thyme and marjoram
dash of hot chili

Lobster with Basil

(Serves four to six)

Raw lobster has firmer flesh and is more juicy than cooked lobster. The taste stays, instead of being boiled away.

Kill the lobster by plunging a knife into the spinal cord. Remove the meat from the shell and run under cold water until it is firm. Cut into bite-size chunks and place meat in dish and squeeze lemon juice over it. Leave to marinate while you prepare the mayonnaise and the seasonings. If possible, leave for an hour. To the mayonnaise add the onion, celery, and basil. Mix well. Remove the lobster meat from the marinade and mix in the dressing. Garnish with slices of tomato and parsley.

3 lobsters
juice of 2 lemons
1 cup eggless mayonnaise (from natural food store)
1 tablespoon finely chopped onion
3 tablespoons coarsely chopped fresh basil
1 tomato
1 teaspoon chopped fresh parsley

Spaghetti and Mushrooms

(Serves two)

Here's another warm meal delight you may prepare without destroying nutrients.

Place spaghetti squash in your oven at the lowest setting (probably warm). Leave the squash until soft and warm (in my oven that's 2½ hours). The slower the vegetable warms, the more food value you are preserving. When the squash is almost done, put the remaining ingredients in your blender for the sauce.

Blend in blender and let sit. Take squash out of oven. Cut squash in half and remove seeds. Pull spaghetti out on plates. Add small amount of hot water to sauce and mix in blender again. Place raw mushrooms on top of spaghetti squash, pour sauce over all.

1 spaghetti squash
Sauce:
tomato paste (from natural food store with no additives)
1 onion
1 clove garlic
oregano
sweet basil
bay leaf
juice of one lemon
freshly ground black pepper
optional: red hot peppers

1/2 pound mushrooms

Stuffed Tomatoes with Shrimp
(Serves four)

Marinate shrimp in lemon juice for three hours, until pink. Hollow out a cavity in each tomato. Salt the cavity. Remove shrimp from the marinade, add the seasonings to mayonnaise, chop the shrimp coarsely, and turn in the sauce. Fill the tomatoes with this mixture, sprinkle the cayenne pepper on top, and decorate with parsley.

1 pound shrimp, washed and shelled
juice of two lemons
4 large, firm tomatoes
1 cup eggless mayonnaise (from natural food store)
1 teaspoon cayenne pepper
sea salt
black pepper, freshly ground
2 teaspoons fresh dill, chopped

Eggplant and Watercress Salad
(Serves four)

Skin and chop the eggplant into small pieces. Salt well and leave for about an hour. Dry off the salt and marinate the eggplant in vinegar for about three hours. Dry and put in salad bowl. Add the watercress, onion, tomato, olives, and herbs. Mix. Prepare sauce vinaigrette by shaking up or stirring together the olive oil, vinegar, a big pinch of powdered mustard, and the crushed garlic. Add to salad, toss, and serve.

1 small eggplant
sea salt
cider vinegar
1 bunch watercress
1 tablespoon Spanish onion, chopped
1 tomato, sliced
1/4 pound black olives
1 teaspoon fresh basil, chopped
1 teaspoon fresh parsley, chopped
4 tablespoons raw olive oil
1 tablespoon apple cider vinegar
powdered mustard
1 garlic clove, crushed

Seviche
(Serves two)

Remove all skin from the fish (your seafood store will do this for you if you request so at the time of purchase) and marinate in lemon juice. Fifteen minutes is enough; overnight, covered in the icebox is terrific! You will notice the fish turning color from the lemon. That is normal — almost a "cooking" process. Cut all the other ingredients into bite-size pieces. Combine.

1 medium fillet of local fish (bluefish is my favorite; any tasty fish will do)
2 medium tomatoes
1 onion (red or white)
3 small chili peppers
1 green pepper
1 teaspoon Tabasco sauce
2 lemons

Potato Delight

(One per person)

Bake potatoes in oven. Mix other ingredients together in blender and use as dressing. Mash into potatoes. Serve as side dish.

*Your favorite potato, yam or
    white
raw olive oil
juice of one lemon
garlic clove*

Sashimi

(Serves two)

Cut the tuna into strips (no problem, as the fish is very tender). Squeeze lemon over fish. Peel the fresh ginger and cut it into thin slices. Serve on a wooden tray.

Once at the dinner table, you may make a kind of "sandwich" out of the fish by placing a slice of tuna in a piece of the seaweed and then adding a piece of ginger and a bit of the hot mustard. Pick up this little roll with chopsticks or your fingers, dip it in the soy sauce, and be delighted.

When I have company, I usually prepare the little rolls in the kitchen and bring them to the table all ready to be dipped in individual dishes of soy sauce placed before each person.

*1 pound raw tuna, or any tasty
    fish
1 lemon
1 package dried seaweed (Nori)
    available at health food store
fresh ginger
hot mustard
soy sauce for dipping*

Tuna Platter

(Serves four)

This is a filling and delicious main meal dish. When you are purchasing tuna, check can labels. You may buy tuna without chemical additives (pyrophosphate) if you shop carefully.

Prepare on a serving platter. Slice avocados and cover the whole platter with them. Slice or chop the onions on top of the avocados. Sprinkle sparingly with cayenne pepper and olive oil. Mix together in a bowl: chopped parsley, green olives, tuna, juice of lemon, and apple cider vinegar. Place on top of avocados and onions. Form tuna mixture into a loaf. This will leave a border of avocado and onion, making a very attractive dish.

*2 cans oil packed tuna fish
2 avocados
1 onion (red or yellow, as you
    prefer)
1 small jar pitted green olives
1 large bunch parsley
1 lemon
1 tablespoon olive oil
2 tablespoons apple cider vinegar
cayenne pepper*

Tofu and Tamari
(Serves two)

This dish may be served warm without cooking, which destroys vitamins. The tofu (bean curd) may be purchased in oriental vegetable stores.

Tamari sauce, a Japanese sauce naturally fermented from soy beans, may be purchased in a natural food store.

Simmer together: tamari sauce, chopped garlic, and honey. Slice the bean curd and place in hot sauce. Serve immediately.

4 cakes tofu
1 cup of tamari sauce
1 clove garlic
1 tablespoon honey

Sweet Potato Surprise
(Serves four)

A colorful dish. When I serve this delicious salad, most people think it's carrots until they taste.

Make a sauce by mixing honey, orange juice, nutmeg, and cinnamon. Combine the rest of the ingredients and top with sauce.

Ellen was particularly taken with this dish. Once she discovered that raw yams were so tasty, she began to eat them in chunks as snacks.

Sauce:
1 teaspoon honey
1/4 cup of orange juice
nutmeg and cinnamon to taste

3 large yams (grated, skin and all)
1/2 head white cabbage (grated)
1 cup raisins (soaked in water for 1/2 hour)
1/4 cup chopped nuts

Avocado and Orange Salad
(Serves four)

Combine the orange juice, orange peel, dried pepper. Add the ginger, seasonings, and carrots. Leave this mixture for an hour at room temperature. Meanwhile soak the raisins. When ready to serve, peel and slice the avocados and squeeze lemon juice over them to prevent them from turning brown. Add the avocados to the bowl with the oil. Add the raisins, mix, season to taste, and serve.

1 cup fresh orange juice
1 teaspoon orange peel, finely grated
1 dried red chili pepper, finely crushed
1 teaspoon fresh ginger, grated
1 cup carrots, grated
2 avocados
3 tablespoons lemon juice
3 tablespoons olive oil
1/2 cup of raisins, soaked in an equal amount of water
sea salt
black pepper, freshly ground

Root Salad

(*Serves two*)

Mix all the ingredients well, add olive oil and lemon juice. Serve on a bed of chopped spinach or lettuce leaves.

1/2 cup carrots
1/2 cup red beets
1/4 cup radishes, grated or finely chopped
1 teaspoon dried basil or tarragon
1 teaspoon honey
1 tablespoon ground horseradish, bottled or fresh

Rice and Okra

(*Serves two*)

Combine tomatoes, soy sauce, and honey in blender or simmer together in pot. Cook brown rice. Steam okra lightly. Serve okra on top of rice and top with sauce. (Do not eat rice more than once a week.)

1 cup brown rice
1/2 pound okra
3 tomatoes
1/2 cup soy or tamari sauce
1 teaspoon honey

Spinach and Sprouts

(*Serves two*)

Wash spinach thoroughly (it tends to hold sand) and tear into bite-size pieces. Add sprouts. Cut sun chokes into chunky pieces (they are very crunchy and nutlike). Sprinkle tarragon over salad and top with a dressing made of apple cider vinegar, olive oil, and a squeeze of lemon.

1 large bunch fresh spinach
1 cup alfalfa sprouts
1 cup mung bean sprouts or soy sprouts
one large Jerusalem artichoke (also known as sun chokes, found in oriental vegetable stores)
1 tablespoon dried tarragon
1 tablespoon apple cider vinegar
4 tablespoons raw olive oil
lemon juice

DESSERTS

Pineapple Boat
(*Serves two*)

Cut the pineapple in half and scoop out the fruit, then cut it into bite-size chunks and mix with orange and grapefruit sections. Pile the fruit mixture back into pineapple shells and top with cardamom-honey dressing.

One pineapple
One orange
One grapefruit

Cardamom-Honey Dressing
(*Serves two*)

Beat the honey with an electric mixer until it is pale and creamy. Gradually beat in the lemon juice and the cardamom seed. Pour over your favorite fruit.

1/2 pint clear honey
2 tablespoons lemon juice
1 tablespoon cardamom seed, cracked

Raw Applesauce
(*Serves two*)

Peel and core the apples. Cut coarse slices and put them in the blender. Add a little cider and blend. Add the lemon juice and seasonings and blend, adding cider until you've reached a consistency that seems right to you.

4 apples, medium size (use juicy apples)
apple cider
juice of 1/2 lemon
dash nutmeg
dash powdered cinnamon
sea salt (to taste)

Cantaloupe Delight

Open the cantaloupe by slicing off a bit of the top. Scoop out the seeds, fill cavity with grapes or strawberries. Fill with port wine and refrigerate. This is a great party dessert!

1 cantaloupe per person
port wine
seedless grapes or strawberries

Prunedate
(*Serves two*)

Blend fruit in cold water to creamy consistency. Blend in hot water and serve over sliced ripe banana.

5 pitted dates (or figs)
3 large pitted prunes
1/2 cup cold water
1/4 cup hot water
2 bananas

Cold Hermint
(*Serves two*)

Blend banana and rejuvelac for 15 seconds. Blend in mint to taste. Place in freezer until time to serve. May also be served at room temperature.

2 super-ripe bananas
1 cup rejuvelac
mint leaves (fresh are preferable, but dried will do)

Cinnamon-Apple Treat
(*One per person*)

Finely grate sweet apples (Delicious are preferable) and season with honey and cinnamon. Top with walnuts.

Paradise Pudding
(*One per person*)

Blend. In minutes, enzyme reactions will produce a most delicious golden pudding. (This is, by the way, a wonderful aid to digestion.)

1 cup carrot juice
1/2 unripe papaya

SNACKS

Most people like a nibble now and then, and why not? The reshaping diet has two categories of snacks: limited and unlimited. You may have two snacks a day.

Limited Snacks

Goat's cheese may be purchased in natural food stores and cheese stores that carry French cheeses. Domestic goat cheeses come from Pennsylvania Dutch country and Wisconsin, and tend to be on the bland side, something like a farmer's cheese. The imported French goat cheeses offer a wide variety of tastes, from bland to sharp and tangy.

Goat's cheese is quite different from cow's cheese and much more compatible with the human digestion. You may have a two-ounce piece by itself, or with a fruit. Goat's cheese spread on a crisp pear is my favorite.

Almonds are delicious, beneficial to your skin, and an allowed snack as long as you *crack them yourself!* Don't buy nuts in packages. Like vegetable juices, their vitamins dissipate. So buy your nuts in the shell and get all the nutrients you deserve. One dozen almonds is your snack.

Almond butter may also be purchased in natural food stores and some grocery stores. Use a low-calorie bran cracker (the brand I use has only 14 calories per cracker). One tablespoon of almond butter, spread thin, will cover three or four crackers. Enjoy. It's delicious. Just stay to the one tablespoon limit.

Unlimited Snacks

Popcorn. Make your own. Buy the kernels in a natural food store, pop with olive oil. Instead of salt, I use kelp powder for seasoning. It's tasty and good for you. Since one cup of popcorn has only 23 calories, you may snack to your heart's delight.

Mung bean sprouts. Crispy, crunchy, and delicious eaten all by themselves. These vitamin-filled taste treats have only 40 calories per quarter pound, so eat all you want.

Fruit. Anytime you're hungry, eat fruit.

Herb teas. There's comfrey and mint, strawberry leaf tea and burdock root tea. Peppermint, Golden Seal, and Chamomile. Hundreds of delicious, healthful, herb teas can be found in any natural food store. Drink them to your heart's delight. Most are wonderful without sweetener, but a bit of honey is allowed.

Chapter 13

The Reshaping Massage

Your skin is a vital organ with a myriad of functions. It is sometimes referred to as the "third kidney" because it is the largest organ of elimination of the body. We also breathe through our skin, absorbing oxygen and releasing carbon dioxide. Some nutrients are absorbed into our body through the skin.

Yet the skin is also our most neglected organ. Men don't often do anything about their skin at all, and while many women will lubricate their face and hands, the other nine-tenths of their body is ignored. A daily dry massage will do the following things: remove dead skin layers and impurities and unclog the pores; stimulate and increase the blood circulation in all underlying tissues, particularly the small blood capillaries; revitalize the eliminative capacity of the skin and stimulate the oil-producing glands; redistribute small fat deposits; stimulate the nerve endings of the skin; rejuvenate the complexion; and, since this is a self-pampering, thoroughly enjoyable task, give you an allover good feeling. In other words, you can't go wrong with a dry massage.

Your massage tool should be a natural bristle brush about the size of your hand, with a long handle that detaches so that you can reach all parts of your body, or a loofah mitt, a coarse natural sponge, or a coarse bath glove of twisted hog's hair. You may also use a regular, inexpensive natural plant-fiber vegetable brush available in any hardware store. Keep your brush clean by washing it in soap and water after every use. Whenever you can, dry it in the sun.

HOW TO DO A DRY MASSAGE

Morning and night are the best times; choose one or both. Begin with the bottoms of your feet, and brush robustly in circles. Cover your entire body in this order: feet, legs, hands, arms, back, abdomen, chest, neck, face.

Take as much pressure from the circling brush as you can without discomfort. You will find that parts of your body differ in tolerance. The most sensitive places are usually the inner thighs, stomach, chest, and face. Some people find their faces too sensitive for this massage. Mine is sensitive, but I do it very gently anyway. Brush and brush; your skin should become warm, rosy, and glowing. Ten minutes is the maximum time you would need to complete your massage, but if you enjoy a longer one, it's perfectly all right. Make sure not to get carried away and brush too hard! You will notice an ashlike dust all over your body when you're through.

As soon as you complete your massage, take an alternating hot and cold shower. If you cannot tolerate the hot and cold shower you may take a normal warm one, but the rejuvenating stimulation on the glandular system and the skin is worth the gritting of your teeth.

Now immediately apply the body lotion described below. It is inexpensive and simple to make. It is a pure product, good for your skin, and you will love the results. The oil will be completely absorbed into your thankful skin, and you need wait only a couple of minutes before you will be able to dress.

A Natural Body Lotion

The oils for this fantastic skin lotion may be purchased at any natural food store. The following formula is enough body oil and moisturizer for a year's supply. You may make less, but keep the proportions of oils the same.

½ cup	Cold pressed sesame oil
½ cup	Cold pressed almond oil
½ cup	Cold pressed avocado oil
¼ cup	Cold pressed or raw olive oil

Blend together and add: 3,000 units of vitamin E from a natural source and 100,000 units of vitamin A from a natural source. (I simply open my vitamin capsules with a pin and add them to the oils.)

You may add a couple of drops of your favorite scent if you wish. Pure perfume is better than cologne. Store in the refrigerator.

Your total cost will be under ten dollars and the improvement in your skin will be immediate from this massage and pure oil combination.

You may just do your brushing massage on the area you are reshaping, but I would rather you stimulate your entire body with this beneficial skin grooming.

Chapter 14

How to Keep Your New Shape

Congratulations are in order! You've worked hard and achieved your goal. Now your mirror image pleases. The lumps are smoothed out, the slack areas well-toned. And, I know you're wondering what's going to happen to this terrific new outline of yours when you stop the reshaping program.

You can never totally stop exercising and retain your present appearance. Whatever area it was that gave you such a problem in the first place will always be the first spot to go if you fall back to old habits. So, in order to keep the problem area in a state of remission, you must adopt a program of maintenance tailored specifically for you.

Each of us is different. The only way to find the perfect sustenance formula for you is to slow down while keeping a careful watch on your body's reactions. Let's take it step by step.

THE FIRST WEEK

If you have a tendency to bounce up and down a few pounds on the weight scale, try not to this first aftermath week. It's difficult to determine what your physical workout requirements are going to be if you're piling on pounds at the same time.

Drop your reshaping workout to three times a week. You've been battling your problem area six or seven times a week. Let's see how your body responds to the reduction of exercise. *Do exactly the same workout.* Don't vary or do less exercise. Keep up the warm-up and stretches. Play at whatever booster you have incorporated into your life-style at least once during this first aftermath week.

On the seventh day, inspect your nude body in a full-length mirror. Is it the same? Check your problem area carefully. If you are satisfied that everything is still in shape, drop to two workouts for the next week and one booster workout.

Examine your outline carefully at the end of the second week. If you're still satisfied with the way you look, this is probably the level for you to stay at. I doubt if you could drop below this number of workouts and stay in good shape.

However, some people are able to maintain a shapely body simply by engaging in their booster sport, *if that booster is aerobic.* Running, swimming, jumping rope, disco dancing, and bicycling all fit into that category. You can give it a try during the third week of aftermath. Stop your reshaping work and do a booster at least twice. Give the exercise its full due; give yourself a really tough workout. Take another look at your figure at the end of this third week. If you've stayed in shape, that's wonderful — just keep at your booster. If your problem is beginning to rear its ugly head, you know that you will always have to work on the spot with your particular reshaper. Perhaps you can do one booster and one reshaping workout per week. Maybe your formula will be one booster and one reshaping workout per week. Maybe your formula will be one booster every week, and one reshaping workout every other week. Experiment until you find the perfect pattern for you.

Your weight will affect the maintenance of your body. If you suddenly put on five pounds, your weak spot will pop. If you stay on the lean side, you're less likely to have to go into full battle again.

If your problem returns, don't get discouraged. An accident or sickness can prevent you from working out for a while. As soon as you are able, however, start your reshaping routine again. You'll snap back quickly. You know how to do the exercises, you know they work, and your body is familiar with the feelings. In no time, you'll be right back in shape.

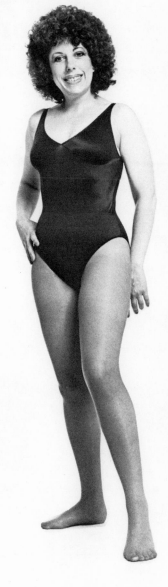

Ellen One Month After

Suggestions for Further Reading

ALLOVER FITNESS

Columbu, Franco and Anita. *Star Bodies*. New York: Clarke Irwin, 1978.

Cooper, Kenneth. *The New Aerobics*. New York: Bantam Books, 1970.

Getchell, Bud. *Physical Fitness*. New York: Wiley, 1976.

Kuntzleman, Charles. *The Exerciser's Handbook*. New York: McKay, 1978.

Lettvin, Maggie. *The Beautiful Machine*. New York: Ballantine Books, 1975.

Lyttle, Richard. *Beginner's Guide to Physical Fitness*. Garden City, N.Y.: Doubleday, 1978.

McKenna, Marylou. *Revitalize Yourself*. New York: Barnes & Noble, 1974.

Morehouse, Lawrence, and Leonard Gross. *Total Fitness*. New York: Simon and Schuster, 1975.

Prudden, Suzy, and Jeffrey Sussman. *Fit for Life*. New York: Macmillan, 1978.

Royal Canadian Air Force Exercise Plans for Physical Fitness. New York: Simon and Schuster, 1970.

GENERAL

Lance, Kathryn. *Getting Strong*. New York: Bobbs-Merrill, 1978.

Ronsard, Nicole. *Cellulite*. New York: Bantam Books, 1975.

Zane, Frank, and Christine. *The Zane Way to a Beautiful Body*. New York: Simon and Schuster, 1979.

Wagner, Kurt, and Gerald Imber. *Beauty by Design.* New York: McGraw-Hill, 1979.

BOOSTERS

Alauz, Michel. *Modern Fencing.* New York: Scribner's, 1975.

Buchholtz, Stan. *Balancing Sport Acrobatics.* New York: Arco Publishing, 1978.

De Carlo, Thomas J. *Balanced Physical Fitness.* New York: Association Press, 1975.

Diagram Group. *Enjoying Gymnastics.* New York: Paddington Press, 1976.

Draeger, Donn. *Classical Bo-Jutsu.* New York. John Wetherhill, 1977.

Draeger, Donn, and Robert Smith. *Asian Fighting Arts.* New York: Berkley Books, 1976.

Filson, Sidney. *How to Protect Yourself and Survive.* New York: Franklin Watts, 1979.

Filson, Sidney, and Claudia Jessup. *Jump Into Shape.* New York: Franklin Watts, 1978.

Fixx, James. *The Complete Book of Running.* New York: Random House, 1977.

Frey & Hoehn. *Beginner's Guide to Swimming.* New York: Doubleday, 1978.

Gaines, Charles. *Pumping Iron.* New York: Simon and Schuster, 1974.

Hittleman, Richard. *Richard Hittleman's 30-Day Yoga Meditation Plan.* New York: Bantam Books, 1970.

Maisel, Edward. *Tai Chi For Health.* New York: Holt, Rinehart & Winston, 1973.

Murry, Jim. *Inside Weight Lifting.* Chicago: Contemporary Books, 1977.

Phelan, Nancy, and Michael Volin. *Sex And Yoga.* New York: Harper & Row, 1967.

Random, Michel. *The Martial Arts.* London: Octopus Books, 1978.

Rossman, Isadore. *Isometrics.* New York: Staven Educational Press, 1976.

ELLEN'S DIET AND RECIPE BOOKS

Airola, Paavo. *How to Get Well.* Phoenix, Arizona: Health Plus Publishers, 1974.

Filson, Sidney, and Claudia Jessup. *Jump Into Shape.* New York: Franklin Watts, 1978.

Gregory, Dick. *Dick Gregory's Natural Diet for Folks Who Eat.* New York: Harper & Row, 1973.

Hodgson, Moira. *The Quick and Easy Raw Food Cookbook.* New York: Grosset & Dunlap, 1977.

Kulvinskas, Viktoras. *Sprout for the Love of Everybody.* Wethersfield, Conn.: Omangod Press, 1977.

Kulvinskas, Viktoras. *Survival into the 21st Century.* Wethersfield, Conn.: Omangod Press, 1978.

Walker, N. W. *Raw Vegetable Juices.* New York: Jove Publications, 1977.

Whyte, Karen Cross. *The Original Diet.* San Francisco: Troubador Press, 1977.